W9-BKP-227

Saint Peter's University Library

Withdrawn

A CHAPTER OF ACCIDENTS

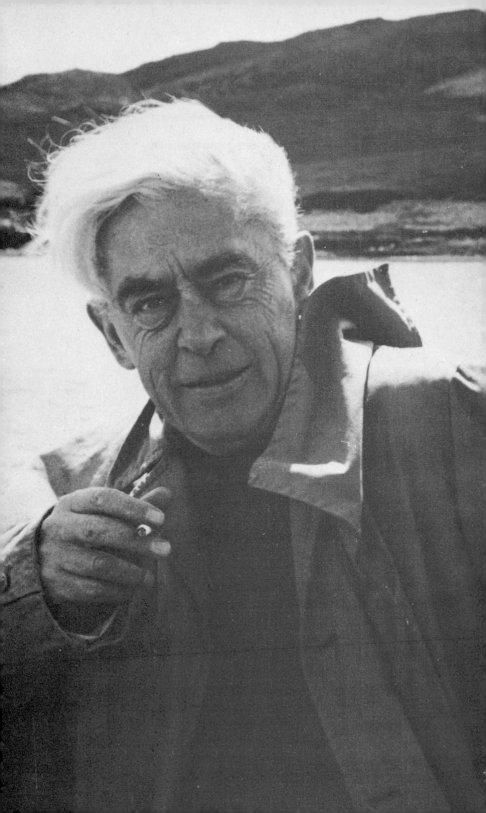

A
CHAPTER
OF ACCIDENTS

by
Goronwy Rees

THE LIBRARY PRESS
New York
1972

Copyright © 1972 by Goronwy Rees

Library of Congress Catalog Card Number:
73-161407

International Standard Book Number:
0-912050-08-X

Printed in the United States of America

FOR
MARGIE
ONCE AGAIN

One

I was born on November 29th, 1909, at Aberystwyth in Cardiganshire, in the early hours of a Monday morning, while my father was away on a preaching engagement which had taken him from home for the weekend. This only happened twelve times a year, and it was thought particularly unfortunate for my mother and myself that I should have been born in my father's absence, as if he could have eased the pains of it both for her and for me.

He was a very intelligent and able man, with a force of character which enabled him to have his own way in most things on which his mind was set. With his natural endowments, he would have achieved success in any walk of life he might have chosen. Originally this was to have been the law, and for this he would have been admirably adapted, intellectually and temperamentally; he was by nature just and fair minded, and his mind would have been at home in its complexities without being led away into abstractions, because he was essentially practical and commonsense in his judgements. He also had a gift of eloquence and persuasiveness which would have served him well before any jury or court of law.

I have no doubt that, if he had followed his original choice, he would have achieved great distinction even in so fiercely competitive a profession, all the more so, perhaps, because to his other gifts he added the essential arts of the politician. He understood the motives which influence men and assemblies and how to manipulate them, he was patient, persistent and flexible in pursuing his own objectives and was always ready for the compromise which would carry a majority with it. His

1

enemies, of whom he had some, would have said that he was a trimmer, but whether this was so or not, it is not often a vice or a virtue which stands in the way of success.

Such qualities eminently fitted my father for that world of politics and the bar to which, in the days when he was young, lack of means was no disqualification. Many young men had started life with worse prospects and fewer abilities than he and had achieved the most eminent positions in the state and at the bar. Some of them I met when I grew up; it never occurred to me that they were superior to my father in either intellectual or practical ability.

But while he was still a boy at the City of London School, something happened to my father which changed the whole course of his life, and therefore, I suppose, my own; or rather, perhaps, it would be true to say that my own existence was merely a subsidiary effect of this intervention of providence. At the age of sixteen my father, like Paul on the road to Damascus, received a call from God, so direct, personal and compelling as to leave no doubt of its authenticity. It was a voice which banished from his mind all thought of worldly ambition and commanded him thenceforward to devote his life to the ministry of the church.

Such a call was of course at that time much less rare than it is now. In those days God often spoke to ambitious young men and changed their lives in a twinkling of an eye, and perhaps it was even less surprising that he should do so to my father than to other young men. For in the middle of the East End of London, with its lurid combination of vice and violence, of squalor and destitution, he had been brought up in a strictly religious and devotional atmosphere, in which the voice of God was heard as frequently and continuously as a television announcer's today, and it is therefore in no way surprising that when

He spoke personally to my father, He should have found a willing and obedient listener.

In one respect, however, His message might be thought to be unusual. When He spoke, though it was within the sound of Bow Bells, it was not in English, or even Cockney, but in Welsh. For in the heart of the East End, my grandfather and my grandmother preserved in almost artificial purity the manners and customs, the religious observances, above all the language of the remote Cardiganshire hills from which they both came. They lived there as Negroes or Pakistanis might today, and in their loyalty to an almost primitive way of life they were strengthened and confirmed by frequent and regular attendance, both on Sundays and weekdays, at the Welsh Methodist chapel which stood within walking distance of their home.

Both my grandfather and my grandmother came of a long line of tenant farmers on the Cardiganshire estate of the Pryses of Gogerddan, whose mansion near Aberystwyth was said to be the oldest inhabited house in Wales. The Pryses administered their estates in the traditionally feckless manner of the Welsh landowner, but they had one distinction which marked them out from most of their class and excluded them from the hatred which the Welsh peasant and farmer felt for most landowners. In politics they were liberal, and indeed the family finances had never recovered from the large expenditure incurred during the nineteenth century in maintaining the liberal interest in Cardiganshire. In a country where every man was a politician, and every working man a liberal, this identity of political interest gave the Pryses a closer hold on the affection of their tenants than was common in Wales in those days. My father used to tell me the story of relations of his from Pembrokeshire, tenants of the

Cawdor estate, who had been evicted from their farm because of their refusal to vote in the conservative interest. They had taken to the road, carrying their belongings with them, and made their way to Cardiganshire to appeal in their distress to my great-uncle. Putting on his Sunday suit and hat, he had interceded on their behalf with Sir Pryse at Gogerddan, who had granted them the lease of one of his farms, partly to spite the Cawdors and partly to reward their fidelity to the good old cause.

But if the Pryses shared the political convictions of their tenants, they looked upon their estates, which extended to over thirty thousand acres of wild hill country, primarily as a means of maintaining the riotous and almost feudal way of life to which they were accustomed, and any measures of improvement were strictly a matter for their tenants, who in any case had little to spare for them out of the meagre income derived from the few sheep and cattle their barren fields would support. Nor, so far as money was concerned, was the landlord much better off. He suffered from a chronic shortage of cash as great as his tenants', and in my grandfather's time, when debts were pressing or the call of pleasure insistent, Sir Pryse would ride out from Gogerddan on a tour of his estates offering reductions in rent to any tenants who happened to have any ready money in the house.

Under such conditions neither tenant nor landlord prospered, so it was natural that my grandfather, being a younger son, should, when he married, obey the iron economic laws which were already depopulating the Welsh countryside and set out for London to make his fortune like many other young Welshmen of the time. His prospects should have been bright. In Wales, Cardiganshire men have an unenviable reputation for thrift, meanness, hypocrisy, money-grubbing and business ability; a "Cardi" is the Aberdonian of Wales, but these qualities had passed my grandfather by, and he was altogether too generous and open-hearted a person to be much of a success in business.

He was not, however, without resources. He had acquired the skill of a stonemason, and my father used to point out to me with pride the roof of the old St Thomas's hospital, which my grandfather had helped to build. His earnings as a stonemason were supplemented by the proceeds of a small dairy which my grandmother managed, for together with their language and their religion they had brought with them to London their traditional attachment to the cattle which had provided them with a living for so many centuries; so that, in the East End, they formed as it were a little pastoral enclosure, where the Bible was always on the table and the cows lowed to be milked in the byre at the back of the shop and occasionally, for their health, were driven out for a blow on Hackney Marshes.

I do not know what commercial ambitions my grandparents cherished when they came to London. Whatever they were, they were not absurd, because, at the end of the last century, the dairy business, like the drapery business, provided many Welsh families with the basis of substantial fortunes. But my grandfather, like his children, and their children after them, lacked commercial sense; he was deficient in that feeling for money which is only given to those who think it more important than anything else, and he was far more interested in his duties as a deacon of the chapel, in the intense political struggles of the period and not least in the varied and turbulent life of the East End streets, than in his business. My grandmother was left very largely to run it herself, and while she did so with moderate competence, she also was too much a child of the country and the chapel to serve Mammon with the exclusive devotion he demands from those on whom he confers large rewards.

Moreover, my grandparents in their own family lacked the support which is very often the reason for the growth of a small into a large business. They were fortunate in having two clever and gifted sons but neither to them nor to their parents did it occur that their future should be devoted to the milk business. My father, when as a boy he accompanied my grandfather in his milk float on his early morning round through the empty streets of the City, was less intent on assisting him than on studying his Greek and Latin texts in preparation for school, while his younger brother had already formed the ambition of becoming a doctor. For both, in their circumstances, the careers they had in mind required a considerable concentration of effort and left them little time to assist in the promoting of my grandfather's business. Nor, indeed, would my grandparents have had it otherwise.

But if my grandparents did not make their fortune, and if their dairy business languished until finally, after my grandfather's death, it died of inanition, it at least provided them with a modest living, threatened neither by poverty nor affluence, sufficient to maintain the standards of independence and respectability which they had brought with them from Wales, and to give them the freedom to pursue those religious and intellectual interests which were also a part of their inheritance. In such matters, at least, they might be said to have prospered; and since my grandfather had a countryman's hospitable nature, as his sons grew up his little house in Hannibal Road became a natural centre for their friends, for young Welsh people whom they knew through the chapel, relations from Wales on a visit to London, medical students from Guy's Hospital whom my uncle brought home, a place of high spirits and eager discussion whose attraction was increased, for young men, by the presence of my father's unmarried younger sister.

Certainly it was a home and a place which offered my father much wider opportunities, in particular as regards schooling, than he would have known on an upland farm; and though in fact he was to spend the greater part of his life in Wales, retracing the steps which had led his parents away from it, it was London that he thought of as his home. He felt that he had been a native of no mean city, and this saved him from the parochialism and provincialism of his native Wales. He remembered that as a boy he had seen the great Mr. Gladstone himself addressing an East End crowd from a brewer's dray, an image that remained vividly impressed on his mind, and this gave him a kind of standard by which he judged men and events in later life.

Most of all, I think, London left him with memories of a kind of happiness, wider, freer, more open to the gales of the world, than he was to know again. No doubt this was partly because, for him, London was bathed in the magic of childhood and youth, and when he died, not long ago, at the age of ninety-six it was to those days that his mind recurred. As his mind wandered in the delirium of his last illness, he told me of the thrill of horror that had passed through the East End at the news of the arrest of the murderer Wainright, with whom my grandfather was slightly acquainted, an imposing figure in frock coat and silk hat, wearing a gold watch and chain, greatly respected in the neighbourhood of the Mile End Road; and of how, when the next morning he walked hand-in-hand with my grandfather through the streets to school, while people gathered on street corners to discuss

7

the sensational news, he felt as if he were walking through a city in which everything was possible, a kind of English Baghdad in which there was no need to be Haroun-el-Rashid to enjoy every conceivable adventure. Dying, it was not of the green fields, the hills and streams of his native country that he babbled but of Stepney Green and the Mile End Road and the East India Docks, as if in those unsalubrious districts there lay buried, like a crock of gold, all the dreams and ambitions he had cherished when he was a boy.

II

It was a natural corollary of my father's decision to preach the gospel that he should enter the ministry of the Presbyterian, or Calvinistic Methodist, Church of Wales, of which the chapel at Jewin which his family attended was a constituent member. The Calvinistic Methodist church was the old, the most respectable and the most prosperous of the many Non-conformist denominations which flourished in Wales. It derived both its theology, which was Augustinian, and its elaborate system of church government, from the rule established by Calvin in Geneva, and to this extremely conservative institution, which in Wales represented what we would now call the Establishment, my father for some sixty-five years devoted all his energies and talents. The very name by which the Calvinistic Methodist connexion was familiarly known, *Yr Hên Gorff*, "The Old Body", shows how far, with the passage of years, it had departed from the spirit of revolt against the established church in which it had its origins.

It was equally natural that, to prepare himself for the ministry, he should return to his native Cardiganshire. For, by a curious succession of historical accidents, there had recently been founded in the remote little seaside

8

town of Aberystwyth the University College of Wales, and side by side with it stood the theological college maintained by the Calvinistic Methodist connexion. The university college had been founded, by public subscription, which was largely made up of the pennies of the Welsh poor, to provide young Welshmen and women with an opportunity for higher education which had hitherto been totally lacking in Wales; it was in many ways the crowning achievement of over a century of agitation to improve the educational standards of the Welsh people. It had the advantage of being cheap and was therefore within my grandparents' limited means; many a country boy arrived at the college laden with a sack of potatoes and a side of bacon which would provide his principal means of subsistence during the coming term.

Having returned to Cardiganshire, it was almost inevitable that my father should repeat a step which all his forefathers had taken before him; that is to say, he fell in love and chose for his future wife, and my mother, the daughter of a small tenant farmer in the same narrow valley in which his parents had been born. It is likely that if he had searched the whole of the world for a wife he could not have made a more fortunate choice.

As for me, I have often wondered at the chance or fatality by which the blood that runs through my veins has been drawn, so far as I know for centuries, from so unmixed a source; and wonder also, sometimes with dismay, what the genetic effects might be of so rarified an heredity. Pharaohs of Egypt could hardly have intermarried more closely than my forebears. This sense of coming from a peculiar people was heightened when as a child I was taken by my father to see the great Professor Fleure, who then held the chair of anthropology at the university. The professor was interested in the shape of my skull, and after close examination and much measurement of frontal lobes and occipital cavities, finally and triumphantly announced, as if I had been some invention or discovery of his own, that it displayed every characteristic of the purest Celto-Iberian stock and none of any other. In England, in later years, I have sometimes felt myself an exile; but so pure a descent almost makes one an exile anywhere, outside an area of about twenty miles square which is almost uninhabited except for one's own relations.

My father, as he confirmed to me later, was too preoccupied with his love for my mother, and also by his interest in radical politics, to devote himself wholeheartedly to his studies at Aberystwyth. He left with a second class degree in classics and then, as a candidate for the ministry, proceeded to Mansfield College, Oxford, where he took a first class in Theology, one of the earliest nonconformists to take an Oxford degree, as the disabilities imposed on them had only been removed by the abolition of the Test Acts as recently as 1878. To have a degree of any kind was something of a rarity in Wales at that time, and, among a people as passionately devoted to education as the Welsh, was a sure passport to public esteem and respect; to have a first class Oxford degree was rather like being elevated to a peerage in a country of philistines like England.

Thus it was again natural and inevitable that, after a brief stay in Pwllheli, in Caernarvonshire, my father should have been summoned to undertake the ministry of *Y Tabernacl*, "The Tabernacle", in Aberystwyth, which was then one of the largest and most prosperous chapels in the gift of the Calvinistic Methodist connexion, and it was thus that I came to be born in Aberystwyth and to spend my childhood there. I have described elsewhere*

* In *A Bundle of Sensations* (Chatto and Windus, 1960)

something of what such a childhood was like, and perhaps it is sufficient to say here that for me they were years of intense happiness. They had all the warmth and security of the womb, only they were also coloured by the green waves and waters of Cardigan Bay, the grey stones of the little town huddled between the sea and the hills, and the streams that poured down in silvery waterfalls and cascades to form the estuary on which the harbour was built. Concealed mysteriously in the depths of Cardigan Bay were the battlements and turrets of the *Cantref Gwaelod*, the lost land of Cockaigne submerged beneath the waves when the drunken Seithenyn omitted to lock its sea gates. Still, on a clear day, the sound of its bells could be heard across the bay, so that one might imagine all the wealth and wonder of that mythical kingdom preserved in its water world beneath the sea.

For a child it was a kind of paradise, drenched in the waters of streams and rivers that might have flowed through Eden. Not far away was the eighteenth-century Gothic mansion which William Johnes had built for himself amid the woods of Hafod and the garden which his little daughter had made for herself beside the waterfall which plunges through them. Coleridge, making an excursion on horseback from Nether Stowey, had once appeared on the skyline overlooking the house and its grounds; surveying as if in a dream its towers and minarets, and the stream cascading beside its water garden, he had absorbed the images which one day were to reappear to him:

> *In Xanadu did Kubla Kahn*
> *A stately pleasure dome decree*
> *Where Alph, the sacred river ran*
> *Through caverns measureless to man*
> *Down to a sunless sea.*

For me the lines have always echoed, as in a sea shell, the music of my childhood; but there were even greater wonders there than in Xanadu. For in the same enchanted circle, beside the ruined monastery of Strata Florida, at Nanteos, the valley of the Nightingale, stood the house which contained the most fabulous and legendary of all treasures, that had given birth to the Matter of Britain: the Holy Grail itself brought there on his miraculous wanderings by Joseph of Arimathea, to become the inspiration of all the poets of Europe and still, in my childhood and even fifty years later, the object of a cult that extended throughout the world. How strange I found it, when I came to read *The Waste Land* and T. S. Eliot's learned references to Miss Jessie Weston, to feel that those myths which had so stimulated his imagination and scholarship, the Grail itself, the Lance and the Wound, the Fisher King, were all part of a world which in my childhood had been as familiar and tangible as the pots and pans in my mother's kitchen.

These were stories which my father told me, but though they enchanted a child's imagination, they lay far apart from my father's interests, which were essentially practical; he lived by works rather than faith. In his years at Aberystwyth his intelligence, his administrative ability, his gift for oratory, made him one to whom, in a small closely knit community, people naturally look for leadership; they earned him the respect, admiration and affection of all who knew him and at a relatively early age gave him an authority unusual in a society in which the principle of gerontocracy was sacrosanct. In the way of life he had chosen, or which had chosen him, the path before him lay smooth and untroubled, and there was no reason why he should not have continued in it with the same happiness as he had begun. All the more so, perhaps, because in the lives of people who, like him, have dedicated themselves to religion, there is a mysterious, irrational element, an X-factor, which removes them from the arena in which worldly success or failure is important.

My father, indeed, had plenty to occupy him; the pastoral care of a large flock, the affairs of the Calvinistic Methodist church, with its elaborate system of ecclesiastical government, the composition of scholarly biblical commentaries, preaching twice on Sunday both in his own and other chapels, where his services were in large demand, the responsibilities of a large and growing family; all this provided an active and interesting life, and I have no doubt that, if left to himself, he would have continued in this course for the rest of his days.

But we are not left to live our own lives and to this rule my father was no exception. The first interference in his orderly, almost predestined course came from an entirely unexpected quarter. In 1921, as a result of the death of the sitting member, a by-election took place in Cardiganshire. Normally, this would have been an event of no more than local interest. Cardiganshire was a stronghold of liberalism, and it was unthinkable that it should be represented in Parliament by anyone but a liberal. But who, in 1921, represented liberalism? The Liberal party led by Herbert Asquith, the true inheritor of the pure Gladstonian tradition in which my father believed, had been annihilated in the general election of 1918 and reduced to a remnant of twenty-seven members in Parliament, and Asquith himself and all its leaders had been defeated. The party had been broken by the devious machinations of the great Welsh statesman and demagogue, Lloyd George, the man who had won the war and now stood at the head of the coalition government, in which one hundred and twenty-seven coalition liberals were outnumbered by three hundred coalition unionists; all alike owed their election to the coupons certifying their loyalty to himself which Lloyd George had issued at the height of his triumph in 1918 as a means of ensuring the return of his government.

In the eyes of many Welshmen, among whom my father would normally have been included, Lloyd George, himself a Welshman and a liberal, was a traitor to the cause with which Wales had hitherto identified its political fortunes, the architect of its defeat and the prisoner of reactionary and imperialist forces which Wales could never look to for any benefits; he had made *il gran rifiuto* and deserved to be consigned to the deepest circle which Hell preserves for treacherous politicians. Besides, for the religious, like my father, moral as well as political considerations were involved; for like everyone else he was aware of the well-substantiated rumours of the Goat's sexual promiscuity, and indeed was well acquainted with a lady who happened to be one of his mistresses at the time. How could a minister of the Gospel, who was also a liberal, hold up such a man to the admiration of his flock?

And now Lloyd George's government, bedevilled by intractable problems of unemployment and industrial unrest, and by its leader's adventures in foreign policy, was tottering to its fall, and Wales prepared to rejoice in it. It had already lost three by-elections in succession, and a further defeat in Cardiganshire might prove a final contribution to the great man's ruin. For a moment the eyes of the world were on Cardiganshire; for Lloyd George was no ordinary politician, he was a world statesman of towering genius and when such a man falls, the world holds its breath. Representatives of the national and the international press descended like a flock of migrating birds on Aberystwyth, drink flowed in the hotels and public houses, and both the Asquithian "Wee-Free" liberals and the Lloyd George liberals organized their forces to consummate or avert the ruin of the Goat. Never since the Midlothian campaign had so tiny an electorate been treated to such a feast of liberal oratory, and there was not a man or woman in the county who was not made aware that on their votes depended the fate of the nation and of the Liberal party.

My father was by nature and tradition intensely interested in politics, and he was as involved as anyone else in the issues which were so inappropriately fought out in Cardiganshire. But he was a politician in more senses than one, and instinct told him that, in his case, the path of wisdom lay in standing aloof from the violent passions provoked by the election. For they were so fierce and so deep that parent was divided against parent, family against family, tribe against tribe; to all the national reasons for bitterness and acrimony were added all the local and personal motives for mutual hatred that exist in a small rural community. The flames of politics were fed by personal and family feuds, by rumour, gossip, malice and slander, until, as the election approached, one might have thought there was not a man in the county who would not gladly have slit his neighbour's throat if it would have had any effect on the result of the poll.

To a person of my father's temperament, essentially reasonable and judicious, not easily given to emotion unless it was a calculated emotion, unsympathetic to the irrational furies of warring Welshmen, with something in him of Asquith's own spirit of compromise and procrastination, a man who liked to weigh his words and the consequences of his actions, it would have been natural to stand aside from the conflict that had broken out in

Cardiganshire and try to moderate passions and reconcile personal animosities so that when at length all was over the belligerents might live together once again in concord and amity. All the more so because the conflict was nowhere more violent than in the bosom of his own congregation, in which, indeed, religious feeling only seemed to give added fury to political differences. In such a situation, pastoral duty required that he should act as a moderator and try to ensure, so far as he could, that the love of Christ should rise superior even to hatred of Lloyd George.

Providence, however, denied him so congenial a role, for which he was so well fitted. The Asquithian candidate in the election was an ageing lawyer from South Wales, who had already represented the party in Parliament but had been one of the victims of the massacre of liberal members in the 1918 election. He had served the party, and Wales, well, and enjoyed the affectionate regard and esteem of his countrymen, of whom only the most bigoted took it amiss that on occasions he was known to over-indulge in alcoholic liquor.

The candidate of the Lloyd George liberals, on the other hand, was a young barrister who had scarcely begun his legal career and was as yet without any claims upon the feelings either of the local electors or of the party at large. He was also the son of a prosperous solicitor in Aberystwyth, who could be depended on to contribute generously to party funds and the expenses of the election, and was a pillar of my father's chapel, its largest single benefactor, and a close personal friend of my father's.

In so closely fought an election, the respect and influence enjoyed by my father in Cardiganshire were factors of not inconsiderable importance. Many would follow where he led, and it was natural that his support was solicited by both parties, and that the Lloyd George candidate's father should press the claims of friendship and gratitude on his son's behalf. Against his instincts, personal, political and pastoral, and with many doubts about the wisdom of his decision, my father yielded to his appeal. What is more, having committed himself to the support of the coalition candidate, he flung himself into the electoral battle with an enthusiasm and effectiveness which surprised even his admirers, shocked others and convinced many that his talents were worthy of some larger arena than Cardiganshire and Calvinistic Methodism. After all, he was a very able man. Like a good advocate, having accepted his brief he made the best of it. He spoke at meetings throughout the county. He could be passionate, eloquent, persuasive, scornful, witty, as the occasion demanded, and was particularly skilful in finding the effective reply to hecklers. When the Asquithians dismissed his candidate contemptuously, because of his youth and inexperience, as a "spring chicken", he delighted his rural audience by replying that he would himself prefer a young bird to an old boiling fowl; it was generally held that he had the best of the exchange, and his candidate's youth ceased to be an election issue.

I say "his" candidate because, even though he doubted the wisdom of his own choice, my father made the cause of Lloyd George and the coalition his own, and while the election campaign lasted he devoted to it all his energies. And if the result proved to be, by the narrowest of majorities, a triumph for the government, it could be and was said that he was largely responsible; in so hard fought a struggle, the formidable qualities he had displayed might well have reversed the result if they had been exerted on the other side.

But alas! victory brought him very little satisfaction, because the consequences he had feared inevitably followed. There were some who regarded him, like Lloyd George himself, as a traitor to liberalism, in Wales then a cause hardly less sacred than that of religion itself. Others said that he, in preferring the worse to the better cause, had put expediency before principle; this criticism came mainly from those who in their own lives would never have dreamed of taking any other course. Some thought that he had been overborne by the influence exerted by Lloyd George and the coalition; some hinted that his motive had been personal ambition and that he had been bribed by who knows what promises of future advancement. What made things worse, in the eyes of his critics, was that his intervention in the election had been so effective. The Welsh admire a victor, but his success always stimulates their secret resentment, and it is the defeated Cato who really wins their hearts.

Worst of all, for my father, such feelings divided even his own congregation and as their shepherd he never again possessed that unchallenged moral and pastoral authority which had previously been his. He had plunged into the muddied waters of politics and had not come out of them unstained; he had shown himself to be, not the servant of truth but a man like other men, with the same passions and weaknesses, a brawler in the market place; his aura had been diminished and in Cardiganshire it would never again have the brightness it once had. Though with time the bitter feelings inspired by the election passed away, for my father things would never be quite the same again. What made it worse for him was his own feeling that, as he confessed to me many years later, he had allowed personal considerations to get the better of what he himself knew to be right.

III

Thus, for my father, the by-election of 1921 cast a certain shadow over his life at Aberystwyth. But another influence also contrived to disturb it and helped to persuade him that after all it would not be right to spend the rest of his days there, as he might otherwise so easily have done. This disturbing influence was, oddly enough, my mother, who though devoted above all to my father's interests and happiness, was also critical enough to feel that life at Aberystwyth made altogether too few demands on him to be entirely for his benefit.

For despite the many claims it made on him, they were not really large enough to place any strain on his abilities, which were quite sufficient for the successful discharge of all his duties without any undue exertion. He was, my mother felt, in danger of becoming too easily satisfied with the part he played in life, and perhaps in this she was right, for there was in my father, as in myself, a certain strain of lethargy, perhaps even of laziness, which made him immune to the kind of inducements which might have appealed to a more ambitious man.

My mother, on the other hand, was compact of energy and activity, and her tiny figure, her large dark eyes, concealed a restless spirit which was never content unless engaged in some occupation, in the home or in the chapel, which taxed all her strength. She was the image of *das ewig Weibliche* which leads men on to larger enterprises than they would have conceived of themselves and provides, by its dissatisfaction with things as they are, a compulsion towards things as they might be.

She had received, at a small boarding school at Towyn, a few miles up the coast from Aberystwyth, a rather better education than most of the farmers' daughters of the class to which she belonged, and a quick mind and an instinctive intellectual curiosity ensured that she made the best use of what she had learned. She was well equipped for the multifarious duties that devolve upon a minister's wife, presiding at the sewing class and the mothers' meeting, teaching in the Sunday school, taking care of the poor and needy, visiting the sick, organizing tea parties, outings, treats, festivals; to all this was added the care of her husband and children and her domestic duties, in which she was assisted by a country girl of a simplicity which was a constant anxiety to my mother because of the temptations offered by what was, in contrast with Martha's native surroundings, the almost metropolitan sophistication of Aberystwyth, whose lights, though dim enough, were almost dazzling compared with the Stygian darkness of night on the mountains. Martha's evenings out were always a period of anxiety for my mother. Who could tell what moral perils she might encounter in the streets and alleys of the town? And indeed her fears were not groundless, for Martha, though slightly slatternly in appearance, was lavish of heart and body and repeatedly found herself pregnant. Except for recurrent and un-explained absences, this seemed to have no effect on her immutable status as maid-of-all-work to the household.

For misfortune, even if combined with immorality, had an irresistible attraction for my mother. She loved all those whom the world has rejected: tramps, gypsies, beggars, lame dogs of every kind, both human and animal, and she loved the needy and the helpless, in particular babies and small children, and it is for this heart overflowing with charity that I most remember her; perhaps because, as the youngest of her children, I was so often its object.

One might have thought that her life, with all its cares and duties, was quite sufficient to absorb all her energies.

And so perhaps for herself it was. But she did not think a small Welsh town gave sufficient scope to my father's abilities and for my brother and myself she cherished the hope of wider educational opportunities than Aberystwyth had to offer. On one of the rare holidays which she and my father were ever able to take together, they had spent a fortnight in Oxford, where my father had shown her the scenes which had meant so much to him in his youth. What she had enjoyed most of all there was to sit and read with him in the gardens of New College. This had appeared to her the most delectable spot in Oxford, perhaps in the whole world and, as my father told me after her death, she had then and there decided that, however unlikely it might seem given our circumstances, I too should sit one day in the same place, not as a visitor, but as of right as an undergraduate of the college.

It was very unlikely that her ambition for me would ever be realized, and it was certainly one of which I, at that time, was entirely unaware. But certainly one of the conditions of achieving it was that I should be given some rather better schooling than was available at Aberystwyth; for we were then still in the days when, for the poorer classes, opportunities of going to Oxford were rare and were the object of the most intense competition.

Thus when the chance came for us to leave Aberystwyth for Cardiff, the after-effects of the great by-election combined with my mother's ambitions to induce my father to accept it, somewhat reluctantly I think on his own behalf, because of the change it would involve in his way of life, but with a sense that he was doing no more than his duty. For his move to Cardiff was again a response to a call from God, as his original return to Wales had been. And in Cardiff there was an excellent boys' grammar school, and to my mother this presented a valuable

21

SAINT PETER'S COLLEGE LIBRARY
JERSEY CITY, NEW JERSEY 07306

stepping stone towards realizing the hopes she had formed for her children.

Fortunately the school agreed to waive, in the case of both my brother and myself, the payment of fees, which, small as they were, would have been an additional strain on my father's purse. And so, in the summer of 1923, when I was thirteen, my father shepherded us down to Cardiff, like mountain sheep moving down from the hills. It was to be many years before I saw Aberystwyth again, and when I did so it was with very different eyes.

IV

My family's move to Cardiff brought about an almost total transformation in the way I had lived until then. To some extent this was true for all my family, but less so, I think, than in my own case, because they were older and had some experience of the world outside Aberystwyth, which for me was still the only world there was. My elder sister was ten years older than I. She had already taken a degree at Aberystwyth, and shortly after we moved took up a teaching post in Barry. My younger sister was looking forward to getting married shortly, and her eyes were exclusively directed towards Briton Ferry, where her future husband, also an ex-student of Aberystwyth was attempting to learn his way in the steel industry.

As for my brother, Cardiff was for him only a brief staging post, at which to matriculate before returning to Aberystwyth, where the university at that time possessed an excellent law school; for he was to be a barrister, as my father had once intended to be, and was already single-mindedly determined to begin his legal studies as quickly as possible. He was a clever boy, and it was normal at that time for Aberystwyth's best law students to proceed to Cambridge after taking their degree.

But for me Cardiff was to be the place in which I spent the whole of my adolescence, as different from childhood as Cardiff itself was from Aberystwyth, and perhaps I associate it with unhappiness both because of the confusion and turbulence of such a phase in one's life and because our migration seemed to bring an end to the warmth and security of the close knit family life we had hitherto enjoyed. It seemed to me that my brother and sisters had grown up and had already entered, or stood at the threshold of, the world of men and women of which I knew nothing, while I was left behind in some grey and mournful limbo of my own, from which all the familiar landmarks of the past had been obliterated. And I think that, in a curious way, my parents had something of the same feeling, with their children growing up and away from them and their own lives so greatly changed from what they had known before.

For my mother especially, who was essentially a country girl, the city of Cardiff always remained as faceless, anonymous and characterless as it was to me; and to her, as to me, the change from the rural atmosphere of Aberystwyth, which was hardly more than a large seaside village, to the great city which Cardiff was by comparison, was a change from community to loneliness. Indeed, the change made itself felt even in our house, for in my later years in Cardiff, when I lived alone with my father and mother for most of the year, it seemed as if the house were empty and deserted, as if we inhabited some melancholy solitude together.

Indeed, everything seemed to contribute to this sense of loss, and for my parents at least it was hard to see what had been gained. The call which had taken my father to Cardiff was an invitation to become the head of what was known as the Forward Movement. This was essentially a missionary enterprise, founded at the end of the nineteenth century, only it was a mission carried out, not among the dark skins which were familiar to us from photographs in reports on Methodist missionary activities in India, but among the heathen of the South Wales coalfield. For the immigrants who poured into the South Wales valleys during the nineteenth century, both from the rest of Wales and from England, formed a very different society from the traditional Welsh rural community on which the Presbyterian Church of Wales was founded. They had either never known the Welsh language or had quickly lost it, and with the language they also lost the religious practices with which it was so intimately bound up. The life of the valleys was savage and turbulent, unblessed by the means of grace, and when the miners emerged out of their underground kingdom into the light of day, they came to the surface like troglodytes out of their caves, not to attend chapel or Sunday school, but to drink and fight, and if they sang hymns it was not to praise God but to celebrate the victory or mourn the defeat of their football teams.

In the eighteenth century, religion had been one of the means by which the Welsh people had been lifted up out of the dark abyss of ignorance, apathy and superstition. The immense growth of population in the South Wales valleys, the birth of a new, raw industrial society, with all the evils that attended it, in the eyes of the Methodist church threatened Wales with a new paganism, a relapse into heathen ways, and called for a new missionary effort to bring the light of religion into the darkness of the pits. The Forward Movement was an attempt to preach the gospel by methods more suited to the passionate temperament of the miners than the staid and respected rituals of the established faith, which from their point of view were

irredeemably "square" and middle class. Visions of hell
fire and of being washed by the blood of the Lamb from
the sins which clung to him like the coal dust he carried
with him out of the pits, were what the miner needed if
he were to turn to God, and the God to whom he turned
had to speak directly to him in words he could understand,
not in the subtle theological terms of the Welsh Calvinists
or through a ministry which had become as sacerdotal as
a bench of bishops. He wanted words that were tinged
with the colour of fire and brimstone and promised him
that, if only he would turn to God, he would be led to
meet his Saviour like a bride prepared for the bridegroom.

It was with such words as these that the Forward
Movement had been intended to call the miners to Jesus
and to such a mission as this that my father now found
himself summoned. My father, though his religious faith
was the most important element in his life and he could
not have lived without it, was essentially a rational man
and for him religion was a part of the life of reason; it
came to him in the terms of a theologian and not of an
Elmer Gantry, and just as he was a liberal in politics so
he was a liberal in theology, for whom religion and reason
were nothing without the other. He distrusted enthusiasm
as much as any eighteenth-century cleric and he had a
respect for the opinions and beliefs of others, an instinctive
delicacy in his dealings with them, which inhibited him
from capturing their souls by violence. I never knew him
to press his own beliefs on me or to try to influence me
in my opinions, though gradually they became so different
from his own that he could hardly fail to regard them as
heretical and even blasphemous; though I was never quite
sure whether this restraint was due to the fact that I was
a hopelessly lost soul or in God's eyes so immutably one
of the elect that it didn't matter what I thought.

He found it difficult to speak the language in which it was thought appropriate to save the souls of the miners, though easy to find his own way to their affection and respect. But there was also a quite different obstacle to the task of winning the miner for God. For by the time my father moved to Cardiff, conditions in South Wales had changed since the Forward Movement had been founded nearly fifty years before. For if, then, religion could have been said to be the only force that thought the miner's soul worth saving, forty years later there was an alternative means of redemption, in the form of socialism, and it was not to the chapel or the mission hall that the miner looked for salvation but to the Labour party and to the local lodge of the South Wales Miners' Federation; while the place of the devil in his cosmology had been usurped by Mr Evan Williams, the chairman of the South Wales Coal Owners' Association.

A man may well turn to God if it's a question of saving his own soul, but personal salvation does not seem an urgent matter if his wife and children are starving. During the long years of the great depression which weighed upon South Wales after the First World War, it might well have seemed to the miners that God had abandoned them in their valleys, and if they were to be saved at all, it would only be by their own efforts; it was not surprising that the evangelical seeds sown by the Forward Movement fell increasingly on barren ground and that the congregations of its mission halls dwindled as conditions in the coalfield deteriorated. It was not in Jesus but in Mr A. J. Cook that the miners hoped to find a saviour; though in the agony of the miners' strike that followed the General Strike of 1926, he hardly proved to be any more effective.

Until that time, indeed, I was hardly aware of the circumstances under which my father laboured to bring the light of the Gospel into the valleys. What I felt more personally and directly were the changes which had taken place in our own domestic life. I had been used to have my father as a continuing presence in the house, where, unless absent on pastoral visits, he worked in his study on his sermons and his commentaries or on the business of the chapel or the methodist connection; one had to lower one's voice or moderate the turmoil of one's games so as not to disturb him and one was always aware that there, in his first-floor study, slightly awesome but always reassuring, he was at work on the mysterious business to which God had called him.

But now he left the house every morning like any business man for his office in the centre of Cardiff, from which he administered the affairs of the fifty or so mission halls which were under his care, or travelled up and down the valleys to visit them. Somehow this diminished him in my eyes; he might have been any company director engaged on the humdrum routine of administration and had lost that essentially personal and individual status of a priest who mediates directly between God and man. And on Sundays it was no longer from his own pulpit that he preached, to his own congregation, every member of which he knew as well as his own family, so that his voice was the voice of a father to them as well as to us, but to strangers in some grim mission hall in a bleak mining village, so that at home his place was empty at table and there was no one to occupy his armchair in which he sat by the fireside to read.

My mother especially missed his presence, day by day and almost minute by minute, for they had lived in much closer and continuous contact than most married couples; and almost as much she missed the cares and duties which she had shared with my father in his ministry to a flock of which she was as much the shepherdess as he the shepherd. It was equally a break with everything she had known till then that the language she heard in the streets was no longer Welsh but English, for the Welsh language was dying in South Wales and even God now spoke in a strange tongue on Sundays. For we also now attended, not the chapel which had hardly been more than an extension of our own home, but one of my father's mission halls in Cardiff and the language of the Forward Movement was English, for the Welsh language was no longer a medium in which to carry the word of God to the masses. The evangelist in South Wales had to preach in English if he was to be understood, just as missionaries in strange lands must use the language of the heathen if he is to touch their hearts.

My mother's life had become lonelier and emptier and perhaps it was because of this as much as for any physical reason that suddenly she, who had always been so active and occupied, seemed to become weaker and frailer; and she had begun to suffer from the heart disease which a few years later was to kill her. She had never seemed old to me, though I was the last born of her children; her love of everything that was young had seemed to make her so herself, and it had never occurred to me that life could continue without her. Now, for the first time, though still with disbelief, I began to realize that one day, in some unimaginable future, it might be possible that she should be taken away from me.

v

I was too young, or too selfish, to understand the changes involved for my parents by moving to Cardiff; or perhaps I was at first too much taken up in my own sense of deprivation, and when that passed too preoccupied by new interests, to notice what was happening to others. For to me at first the loss of my childhood world, so tiny and circumscribed, yet somehow open to all the seas and skies of the world, was a shock that was almost traumatic. I felt as if I had been cast out of paradise, and with a sense not of loss only but of guilt, as if somehow it was my own fault. Most of all I missed a certain quality of perception which, in my childhood, had seemed to make everything at once familiar and magical and now, under the shock of removal to the city, seemed to wither away like some fabulous plant that would only blossom in its native soil.

For my first, yet enduring impression was of the unrelieved ugliness of the city, of its long grey streets and the monotonously repeated vistas of identical terrace houses, the muddy complexion of its stones and the hideously flaring red and orange of its bricks that inflicted themselves on one's sight like a wound. They affected one's eyes like some painful ailment, as if they had been rubbed sore by seeing. To me this world which man had built for himself seemed utterly inhuman, hostile to all the innumerable responses of the nerves and the senses, while the natural world which pressed so closely upon one in Aberystwyth had been so perfectly attuned to every infinitesimal impulse that it seemed to fit one like a glove.

I had never been to a city of any size before and its wastes of brick and mortar weighed upon me with a dull sense of oppression that was like a physical pain. It was years before I realized that even city landscapes can have their own beauty and certainly there was little of this to be seen in Cardiff. Walking or cycling to school through the long grey tunnel of Mackintosh Place in which every grey little house faithfully reproduced the hideousness of its neighbour, or down the tramlines of the City Road where neither the shops nor the objects offered for sale in them had any quality or virtue except the grimmest utility, I would feel a sense of leaden hopelessness, as if these streets stretched on into infinity and there would never be any escape from them, mathematically parallel lines projecting the city and its inhabitants in an endless future of which every moment was nothing but the exact and senseless repetition of what came before and after it. Sometimes I could hardly believe that the sea, blue, smiling, and welcoming, was not awaiting round the corner and it was with a sense of doom, as of a condemned man, that I realized there lay before me only another monotonous perspective of the no-man's-land of the city.

In those first years in Cardiff I began to feel, for the first time, that destructive sense of depression which reduces the whole of life to a uniform monochrome and transforms every impulse to thought or action into the meaningless reflex of a mechanical puppet. It is a sense which has frequently recurred to me in later years; for those who feel it, it is so acute that it eats like acid into the texture of life, so that it falls away from one in shreds and tatters, like some threadbare garment which has worn so thin that it can no longer hold together. And whether or not it was the fact of our removal that induced my depression at that time, or whether it had its roots in deeper causes, it is true that for a year or two I underwent some mysterious form of sea-change, some hidden revolution in the depths of the self, which coloured all my experiences and made them so dark, confused, and fragmentary that they hardly seemed to be mine at all.

We cannot truly see what is happening in the darkest recesses of the self, nor can memory accurately reproduce what is so fitfully and partially perceived. Perhaps it would

be better simply to say that for a time I felt totally disorientated in the new world we had entered, stumbling
about in it awkwardly and childishly as if my limbs were
no longer under my own control and my feet no longer
knew where they were carrying me.

For at first it was a world of strangers, and the boys I
met in my new school seemed to me so different from
those I had known before that they hardly seemed to
belong to the same race. And indeed to a large extent they
did not, because Cardiff is as much an English as a Welsh
city, a mongrel border town in which the Welsh strain
has been so diluted as to produce a far more variegated
social pattern than I was accustomed to. But to me at least
the boys in my school were alike in that they were all
different from me, and in particular in being, or appearing,
infinitely more mature and sophisticated, with the sharper
wits and quicker intelligence of the town dweller, and the
adaptability that came of living in a more complicated
social structure than Cardiganshire had to offer. They
laughed at my country accent, and even more at the
curious garments my mother had constructed for me
from a cast-off suit of one of my uncles, with trousers that
hung well below the knee to allow for growth and a high
buttoned jacket that might have been fashionable today
but then had more than a touch of the grotesque. I had
been proud of the suit when I first wore it, because the
material was excellent and it had been tailored by mother's
own hands, but now I quickly and shamefully realized
that in the town it made me an object of ridicule and
mockery.

So perhaps it was not surprising that for some time
I found it difficult to adapt myself to my new school. My
brother, who had a better character and a more single-
minded purpose than I, appeared to escape such

difficulties and continued to achieve the same excellent academic results as ever; I on the other hand failed lamentably. In Aberystwyth I had been thought a bright boy, as became the son of my father; but in Cardiff I tended towards the bottom of my form with such consistency that my mother's ambitions for me seemed to be more absurd than ever. Indeed, even she began to lose faith, and when, at the end of my second year in the High School, I returned home with a report which was more than usually unsatisfactory, and my brother with one which was, by contrast, of almost dazzling achievement, my mother burst into tears and confessed that she could not see what was to become of me. "If you go on like this", she said amid her tears, "you'll never be anything better than a bank clerk."

A bank clerk! It was a curious threat, for in those days when any form of employment was hard to come by in South Wales, to be a bank clerk might seem to promise an enviable future to almost any boy, secure, relatively well paid by our modest standards, and with the assurance of an eminently respectable social status. Yet my mother was right, and to me her words were words of doom; for to me as to my mother they signified a life of dull-minded devotion to commerce and the worship of Mammon, unilluminated by any higher interest, and neither she nor I thought that was a life worth living. As for me, I had already formed a quite different conception of what my life was to be, though if my mother had known of it she might have been no less dismayed than by the future with which she had threatened me. For I had already decided that by some means or other I would become a writer, though how this was to be achieved I could not guess, nor had I any reason for thinking that I possessed any of the talents it would require. In my eyes, there could be nothing more incompatible with a writer's life than the to me infinitely dreary calculations of profit and loss which I supposed to be the exclusive occupation of a banker.

But however vague my ideas of how I was to satisfy my literary ambitions, or even, indeed, of what it really means to be a writer, they were already sufficiently clear to make me face the choice which presents itself to every young Welshman with the same heritage and upbringing as myself; it was the choice of whether to write in English or Welsh, either of which, at that time, would still have been possible to me. Nor was this simply a choice between two languages, entailing no further consequences. For every language has its own particular genius, and the language which one writes and speaks also very largely dictates what one thinks and what one feels. There are things that can be said in Welsh that cannot be said in English, just as there are things which can be said in English that cannot be said in Welsh, and in choosing a language one is not only choosing a vocabulary and a syntax but what one can say with them. Otherwise, the problem of translation would not remain the almost insoluble one that it is.

Today I feel surprised that, given my attachment to the scenes and language of my childhood, I should have made the choice so easily, almost without thinking, as if, for me at least, no choice was really necessary. Indeed, I can distinctly remember the moment when I made it. When I was fifteen, my Welsh master in school, himself a minor poet in his own language, asked me what I wished to be when I grew up. I answered that I wished to be a writer. "In Welsh or in English?" he asked; and went on to explain that a writer in English, which is a universal language, must expect to meet the most intense competition, which only the most talented could hope to survive, while in Wales, which has no professional writers and all are amateurs, the field was narrowly confined, and given any talent at all I could hardly fail to make some name for myself.

The advice was well meant, and I have no doubt that my Welsh master may well have been in the right; certainly he had my best interests at heart. But it was an unfortunate argument to use to a boy, and it was all the less attractive in the mouth of a patriotic Welshman. I have no doubt that, in a sense, and without knowing it, I turned my back upon Wales at that moment and since then I have had no reason to regret it. For literature then was already becoming for me something that is more important than nationality, a means of release from a way of life that had begun to seem cramped and constrained, and the key to some wider world than Wales had to offer. It was as if, in choosing the language of my childhood, I should have chosen to remain a child for ever, and this is something Welshmen often do. As for me, I felt that in leaving Cardiganshire I had left the happiness of childhood behind and, even if I wished, could not have it again. The trouble was, I suppose, that I wanted to grow up and felt that I could not do it in Welsh.

It was not ambition that made me want to be a writer, nor any belief in my literary talents, for this I have always lacked. It was the thought that outside there lay a wider world in which there were larger issues at stake than those which obsessed us in the narrow circle in which I had been brought up, where everything seemed certain and predictable and one might live and die without encountering more than a very few of the infinite varieties of human experience. It wasn't that one wanted to compete with others; one wanted to compete with oneself and see what one was capable of, like a gambler who will never leave the table until he has lost everything.

It is difficult now to unravel the labyrinthine workings of a boy's mind, partly because at the time one was largely unaware of one's motives and even now they have hardly become more clear. But somehow I date to this period, somewhere between my fifteenth and sixteenth year, a kind of awakening out of the mood of depression, compounded of nostalgia and apathy, into which I was thrown by my parents' move to Cardiff.

It helped to save me, at a time when I myself doubted whether I was worth saving, that my mother proved to be right in her instinct that, educationally at least, our migration to Cardiff would prove to be for my good. The High School at Cardiff, at the time when I attended it, between 1923 and 1928, was indeed an excellent one, so good indeed that for me it still represents the ideal of what a school should be, and I still sometimes wonder at my good fortune in attending it. In the classics, in mathematics, in history and in English we were taught by men of quite exceptional ability and qualifications; my history master later held a university chair and became a Welsh historian of the greatest distinction.

I have often wondered since why men of such high intellectual capacity should have been content to devote themselves to the ungrateful task of teaching a somewhat rough and unruly set of boys. Partly, I suppose, it was because at that time schoolmastering as a profession provided a security and, especially in Wales, a social status which, alas, it no longer does, and a salary envied by many at a time and place where unemployment was a constant threat. But it was also because those men felt a genuine compulsion to impart their knowledge and their own high intellectual standards to their pupils, and this gave to their teaching a kind of urgency and passion which made education both an inspiration and a pleasure.

Most of all they were marvellously responsive to any sign of talent or ability and were wonderfully generous in the pains they took to foster it. They talked to one as if one were as adult and intelligent as they were; they answered one's questions and discussed the answers as if everything they said was only a basis for further questions; they lent one books and encouraged one's own interests; somehow one felt that the distinction between master and pupil ceased to have any importance compared with what was shared between them.

In all this we were the beneficiaries; and all the more because the school combined with its high standard of teaching an admirable freedom in matters of discipline, and for me, who was apt to resent any form of restraint, this was particularly fortunate. The headmaster, who looked rather more like a Prussian officer of the old school than a teacher, was himself only a moderate scholar, though he had a passion for the classics; but he had something which is even more valuable than scholarship in a schoolmaster, which was a deep and sincere respect for the individuality of every boy in his care, whether clever or stupid, docile or rebellious. There was little attempt at what is known as "character forming" and, outside their work, boys were left to become very much what they wanted to be. For the headmaster and his staff had grasped the essential truth that the larger part of life lies outside the walls of a school, and especially a day school like ours, and consciously or unconsciously they drew the conclusion that they could best serve their pupils by concentrating on the one function they were in a position to discharge most effectively; that is to say, the task of inculcating the highest intellectual standards which their pupils were capable of absorbing and of providing them with the basis of knowledge which they would require if they were to achieve either success or pleasure in life.

And curiously enough, by doing so they achieved, though by indirection, a far greater moral influence than if they had consciously attempted to shape and form that most elusive and amorphous of all natural phenomena, the character of an adolescent boy. For the process of learning, at any stage above the most elementary, has a moral value of its own, in which respect for truth is the greatest ingredient, and even boys are capable of absorbing it when properly taught; it is a kind of uncovenanted grace which is added to the other advantages and pleasures of learning. And perhaps something of this civilizing influence did make itself felt in the school. We were on the whole a rough lot, mostly of the lower middle class, and most of us were passionately addicted to Rugby football, which is not the most civilizing of pastimes; but there was very little of the cruelty or brutality, physical or mental, to which boys sometimes subject each other, or are subjected to by their teachers. If this was so, it was largely because of the staff, who were themselves humane and civilized men and were too interested in their teaching to have time to waste on the kind of petty persecution which sometimes goes by the name of discipline.

I do not know what kind of verdict would be passed on the school if it were judged by modern educational standards. I imagine it might be said that it was too insistent on formal academic instruction, that it took things like examinations very seriously and prided itself on its academic record; yet in fact the education it gave was surprisingly wide and varied, and opened a boy's eyes to much broader intellectual vistas than the ordinary curriculum normally provides. Even today I am still surprised that our history master should have thought it worth while to include in his course a class in Plato's *Republic*, which was in fact an excellent introduction to philosophy; or that our English master should take me to his home to show me his excellent library and especially his fine editions of Blake and Donne, and by doing so inspire a lifelong devotion to both poets. He had once been a minor poet himself but was now a bibliophile and he did not care for the turn which modern poetry was taking; but when I, having found *The Waste Land* on the shelves of the Cardiff Public Library, announced my admiration of T. S. Eliot, he asked me to his home to explain to himself and a friend what were then still the mysteries of that poem. I do not know that I, a schoolboy with even less knowledge of life than of literature, made much of my job of my exposition; but I do know that, in my youthful and incoherent enthusiasm, I was listened to with as much interest and respect as if I had been Mr Eliot himself, and that at the end of a long evening's discussion of what the poem meant and of what it portended in the development of English poetry, I had learned far more than either of my sympathetic listeners.

Under such circumstances, learning becomes a pleasure and certainly it was largely due to the kind of education I received at school that after a time I began to struggle out of the mood of bewilderment and incomprehension induced by our moving to Cardiff, and that the acute sense of having lost the world of my childhood gradually diminished and gave way to the hope that perhaps, somewhere, life might again have to offer the same infinite possibilities which surrounded me as a child. Most boys, I think, in the process of growing up, suffer the same sense of transition from one world to another and it is only accident which decides with what particular places or experiences it is identified, and accident also which decides with what degree of pain or difficulty the transition is made, or indeed whether it is made at all. For there are some unfortunate ones for whom the attachments of childhood are never overcome, and some for whom the pain and confusion of its passing never wholly cease, so that they remain for ever irretrievably fixed in a past which has never been transcended.

As for me, I was lucky, so much so indeed that for many years, until experience taught me otherwise, I was accustomed to think of myself as a favoured child of fortune. I was lucky in finding people who gave me a hand across the bridge which, poised so precariously above an abyss of doubts, confusions and uncertainties, leads from childhood to manhood. It was not only they who made the difference; but they helped as it were to dispel the mist which fogged my sight, so that at moments one might at least catch a glimpse of what the future might be. Certainly, so far as education was concerned, their encouragement was so far effective that my academic performance after a time began to inspire a hope that my mother's ambitions for me were not, after all, quite so absurd as they had once seemed. From about my sixteenth year, it began to be taken for granted that I should sit for a scholarship to Oxford, and preferably, because of the pleasure the gardens had once given my mother, to New College.

The trouble was that so simple and, as it seemed, so obvious a choice, did not altogether recommend itself to me. It would be difficult to explain my reluctance to follow my parents' and my schoolmasters' choice, because partly at least they coincided with my own. Perhaps it was simply that they were my parents and schoolmasters and therefore in my eyes incapacitated by age and experience from giving any advice which could have any possible relevance to me. I realized, of course, that they wished to do their best for me and that it was my own good they had at heart; but after all, who were they to know what was best for anyone as peculiar as myself. By peculiar I did not mean anything that was in any way flattering to me. It was only that I recognized in myself, however obscurely, something which would make it impossible for me to live or want to live as they did.

It was part of the trouble that I really knew nothing about what either Oxford or Cambridge was like, and the little that I did know did not altogether recommend them to me. There were a few older boys from the school who had already preceded me there, for though in those days it was difficult and rare for any secondary school children to attend either of the older universities, there was one sure way to secure both admission and the necessary financial resources. This was Rugby football. It is a peculiar reflection of both the economic and the educational environment of the time that football could protect a poor boy against his disadvantages in either respect. It could open a way to Oxford or Cambridge because of the immense importance which its colleges, and the English ruling class of which they were the cradle, still attached to playing football, and there was always some form of financial assistance available to anyone who played Rugby football well enough to be a potential blue or international.

In the same way, he was protected against the threat of unemployment, which was a very real one in the valleys, because he could always turn professional and go to the Northern League. Wakefield and Balliol were equally open to a boy who was moderately good at his work and a very good scrum half. In later years I knew a

miner's son who having both won a scholarship and been
offered a contract by Huddersfield, was tempted to choose
the latter because it would allow him to contribute to the
support of his family, of which the father and his three
brothers were all unemployed. In fact, he chose the
scholarship and eventually became a professor but ever
after felt he had taken the selfish course.

None of the boys from my school who went up to the
ancient universities on the strength of their athletic
promise was stupid; they were above rather than below
the standards required for admission in those days. But
what they were in the first place was superb footballers,
and when they returned to Cardiff in the vacations they
had adopted all the physical and mental attributes of the
typical university athlete of the time, the hearty bonhomie,
the Philistine outlook, the public school slang. They had
become almost a caricature of the type; in their Oxford
bags, their tweed caps, their scarves and blazers, they
appeared to us who were still at school as some kind of
athletic *jeunesse dorée* and it seemed to me that if this was
all the university could do for them, it could not do very
much for me.

On the other hand, I had seen some of the almost tragic
cases produced by the then fierce competition for the few
scholarships available to those who had no ability to kick
a football; clever and poor boys, inspired by ambition, who
had set their hearts on proceeding to the older universities
but had never quite succeeded in amassing the financial
means to do so, and so had stayed on in school year after
year to repeat the same dreary cycle of scholarship
examinations which, even if sheer persistence eventually
brought them success, had already broken their hearts and
their spirits. There seemed to me something both cruel
and pathetic in such endeavours and they did nothing

to encourage me to enrol in what was fundamentally a harsh and inequitable system. For I was already a socialist, or thought myself one, and in 1926 had already had my first view of industrial and civil strife, when the stalwart members of the Glamorgan constabulary had stood shoulder to shoulder against the sullen crowds in the streets of Cardiff and mounted police had charged them in St. John's Square. Nor had my affection for either Oxford or Cambridge been increased by the sports-jacketed undergraduates who had descended upon us to assist in maintaining the public services and in breaking the threat to their way of life represented by miners who, up in the valleys, had emerged from their underground kingdom to claim a share of the wealth which had been so generously bestowed upon these oafish and arrogant youths.

Oxford seemed to me the very heart of the English class system, of what we had not yet learned to call the Establishment, and, as such, to be entirely alien to the romantic dreams which had begun to haunt my imagination. For Oxford, in my prejudiced view, not merely represented the opposite of what I felt to be the just and natural order of things; what was even worse, it seemed to me the enemy of those affections of the heart and those flights of the mind which are both the source and the material of art.

For it was such matters that, by the time I was in the sixth form, had begun to fill my mind and take the place of what had hitherto been an obsession with Rugby football. And once again my own instincts and inclinations were encouraged by the atmosphere which prevailed in my school. It was one of the headmaster's firm beliefs that by the time they entered the sixth form boys were in danger of having a surfeit of formal instruction, and of working to the demands of a rigid curriculum, and that the time had come for them to find out for themselves where their real interests lay. So that for a year we were left very much to ourselves, to do what we liked or even to do nothing at all, following no particular curriculum and with the easiest possible schedule of prescribed work. It was the principle of the Sabbatical year applied to schoolboys, and it seemed to work with the greatest possible success. Nothing could have been more unlike the pressure exerted today on an aspiring schoolboy, the grim insistence on specialization and all its attendant evils, the *ewige Widerkehr* of the examination system, and for myself I still remain grateful for that year of idleness and freedom suddenly granted one in the middle of the long process of education.

I say idleness and freedom because that was how it appeared to me. It would be truer to say that for a year nothing was asked of one which one did not choose for oneself. My brother used the same year to take the London Matriculation examination, instead of the normal Higher School Certificate, because it allowed him to go to the university a year earlier than usual. I used it to indulge what has become an almost obsessive passion for literature and in trying to penetrate its secrets for myself. My English master's fine editions had already introduced me to Blake, who has remained one of the abiding interests of my life, and through reading Edwin J. Ellis's *The Real Blake* and his and Yeats' commentary on Blake's mystical works, I came to read Yeats' own poetry. When a boy is started on a course of reading like this, there is no knowing where it may lead him; it is an addiction as powerful and compulsive as drugs. In my own case, Yeats led me on to read Arthur Symons, to struggle, with the aid of my schoolboy French and pocket dictionary, to make sense of the French symbolist poets and to try to find some meaning in Yeats's combination of Celtic mythology and cabbalistic lore. I placed roses under my pillow at night so that I might dream of the Sacred Rose, which is the rose of all the world, and believed that, if only I concentrated enough, I would hear the shields and spears clashing in the Valley of the Black Pig.

Such ideas make a heady draught for a boy of sixteen and they drove me into ways which were no doubt absurd but which I have never regretted. For I was possessed by a state of exaltation which made me believe that in such books I might, with sufficient effort on my part, seize hold of the key to the secrets of the universe; they were not only literature to me, they were the deepest manifestations of life itself. The chief source on which this exaltation fed was nothing more esoteric than the open shelves of the Cardiff Public Library, where as if drawn by some invisible thread, like that one which led Theseus to the Minotaur, each book seemed to direct me to another so that I became engulfed in some strange universe of discourse, infinitely remote yet infinitely real, whose secret paths and tortuous ways were only revealed to the adept.

On Saturday nights in winter, after playing football for the school in the afternoon, I would walk through Cardiff's streets, crowded with miners come down from the valleys to watch the match at Cardiff Arms Park and their wives enjoying the city's sights, and through the market near St. John's Church where under their garish lights the stalls displayed the hot meat pies and black puddings and larva bread which were then the delicacies of the poor. The lights, the crowds, the drunks lurching out of the pubs, the girls waiting to be picked up made of Cardiff something entirely different from its drab every day; it was like walking on to the stage of a theatre in which everything has suddenly become much larger and brighter than life. I was already bemused and dazzled when I entered the cool mock-Gothic spaces of the library, but what lay within was no less enthralling than the scenes outside, and for a moment, in the entrance hall, I paused, almost dizzily poised between the real world and that other one which lay embalmed within the covers of the thousands of books that filled the library's shelves.

Yet to me in those days there was no real distinction between the two, and my experience of the world was so small that I saw the people in the street with the same eyes with which I absorbed the treasures that lay on the printed page. Chance alone first made me lay my hand on *The Waste Land*, and this led me to *The Sacred Wood*, and *The Sacred Wood* to the Elizabethan dramatists, and they in turn to the metaphysical poets. One day my hand fell on a book that was strange to me, *Centuries of Meditation*, by Thomas Traherne, and on the first page where I opened it I read: "The corn was immortal wheat, which never should be reaped nor was ever sown. I had thought that it had stood from everlasting to everlasting. The dust and stones of the street were as precious as gold; the gates were at first the end of the world. The green trees when I saw them first through one of the gates transported and ravished me, their sweetness and unusual beauty made my heart so leap, and almost mad with ecstasy, they were such strange and wonderful things. The Men! O what venerable and reverend creatures did the aged seem! Immortal Cherubims! And young men glittering and sparkling Angels, and maids strange seraphic pieces of life and beauty! Boys and girls tumbling in the street, and playing, were moving jewels. I knew not that they were born or should die; but all things abided eternally as they were in their proper places. Eternity was manifest in the Light of Day and something infinite behind everything appeared; which talked with my expectation and moved my desire."

How can one explain why this should have struck one with the force of a revelation, not by its beauty only, but as an expression of objective truth, which applied as much to the streets outside the library as to anywhere else in the world. I added it, like some jewel of infinite worth, to the personal treasury I had amassed out of my reading, a kind of Aladdin's cave in which was piled a jumbled and hetero-geneous hoard of ideas not only from Blake and Yeats and the French symbolists and Eliot, but also from *The Golden Bough* and Sir John Rhys's *Celtic Pantheon*, which was on my father's bookshelves at home and, even more incon-gruously, Wyndham Lewis's *Time and Western Man*. For in those days everything seemed to lead on to every-thing else, and in these universal lines of communication I felt as if I had discovered some secret wisdom which enabled me to interpret the world as it really is, if we only had the eyes to see it; and as I walked home from the library, weighed down by a pile of books bound together by a leather strap (for I had impounded all my family's library tickets) the streets of Cardiff, gaudily lit in the centre and gradually growing dark and deserted as one penetrated into the suburbs, were not populated by men and women or built of bricks and mortar but had become a theatre for figures and images out of the *Spiritus Mundi*, which reveals itself through that secret system of corres-pondences which only the initiated can decipher.

The mysterious workings of chance led to another discovery. One of the few social centres for the ordinary citizens of Cardiff, except, of course, for public houses,

was the café attached to the Capitol Cinema where people
in search of some distraction from the grim tedium of
lower middle class provincial life could sit and drink
coffee, and eat egg and chips, amid what seemed then the
grandiose surroundings of this recently built super
cinema. There my brother one night had fallen into conversation with a stranger, a slight dark thin man, with the
high complexion of the tubercular but with a gaiety and
vivacity which were enhanced by his Dublin accent. His
name was Nagel, and he was an actor from the Abbey
Theatre, forced into his retirement by his complaint and
living in Cardiff because its air was said to be good for it,
though it would be hard to say what recuperative powers
he drew from the coal black waters of the river Taff,
flowing between its muddy banks past the particularly
sordid actors' lodgings which he occupied on its embank-
ment; unless, perhaps, the river reminded him of the
Liffey.

My brother struck up an acquaintance with him, and
before he left Cardiff for the university, introduced me
to him, believing, rightly, that he would appeal to my
literary tastes. For his conversation was full of reminiscences of the Abbey Theatre, of Moore and Gogarty
and Synge, in whose plays he had appeared. He had even
seen and heard and known Yeats himself, which for me
was if he had met Blake, and had lived in Paris and had
acted on tour in the United States.

Nagel was the first person I had ever known for whom
literature did not come out of books but out of life, and
this seemed to give another dimension to the dreams and
fantasies that filled my mind, as if, poor and ill as he was,
his mere existence seemed to endow them with flesh and
blood. But he opened my mind to vistas and possibilities
to which until then my only access had been through

books, and he spoke of writing and writers as if they were not something alien and exotic but as natural and familiar as the air one breathed, and for that I owe him a debt which I was never able to repay, because soon after I left school his condition deteriorated and he died in a sanatorium to which he had been removed high up on the Brecon Beacons.

His large and general claim upon my gratitude included one obligation which was particularly heavy. One evening, as we sat over our coffee cups in the café, he placed upon the table a thick volume covered in brown paper so that I could not read its title. I instinctively reached out to take it but he placed his hand over it, as if he could scarcely bear to let it out of his possession.

"What is it?" I asked.

"It's a book," he said.

"I can see that," I said rather rudely; "but why so much fuss about it?"

"It's by the greatest writer now alive," he said, and opening it showed me the title page: *Ulysses*, by James Joyce.

It was a copy of the first edition printed by Sylvia Beach in Paris. In those days, *Ulysses* was still banned by the Home Office, copies of it were difficult to obtain for most people, and except in the very smallest circles it had not yet established itself as the masterpiece which it is. As for me, for all my reading I had never heard of it, and regarded with some scepticism what I took to be Nagel's extravagent claims for the author, who, he explained, was a Dubliner like himself; it was as if I had claimed that one of our obscure neighbours in Roath Park was a great writer. But he lent me the book, and for a few weeks I was plunged into a world, a city and a language that were not like anything I had ever known before. I do not know that I understood even a tenth of what I read, but somehow, through the kind of empathy which enables the young, in their reading, to penetrate the secret of what they do not understand, the book became a part of me, and Buck Mulligan beside the snot green sea, and Mr Bloom and Stephen Daedalus the kind of friends who remain beside one throughout one's life.

I even took the book to school with me to read in my spare time, and being discovered doing so by the head-master was beaten for introducing pornography into the school; even his tolerance did not extend to *Ulysses*. It was the second of the only two times I was ever beaten at school. My father, on the other hand, after looking through the book one day when I had left it lying in his study, merely said: "There seems to be a lot of obscenity in this book," and handed it back to me with distaste indeed, but with no further attempt to interfere with my choice of literature.

VI

The truth is, I think, that during much of my last years in Cardiff I was on a trip quite as delirious and hallucinatory as any recommended by Dr Timothy Leary, only its motive power was provided by literature and not by drugs. But there are cases in which the one can be quite as powerful as the other. The breath-taking flights into the unknown, the precipitous plunge into mysterious caverns of the imagination, were as dizzy as any psychedelic addict's; one's eyes were dazzled, one's ears roared with the boom of undiscovered oceans, the world was a storehouse of cryptic messages which only awaited one's attention to unlock their meaning. It was as if one monitored the communication system of an invisible universe, infinitely distant and yet so close that one had only to lift a hand to touch it, and at times so vividly and intensely seen, heard, felt, smelled that the senses became confounded and bemused.

To me this world to which I could give no name was at times so real and palpable that it blotted out my every-day experiences, the people who surrounded me seemed no more than tenuous ghosts and I myself had no more individual existence than a tree or a stone. One could quite truthfully say, in modern jargon, that I was both disorientated and alienated; every day

> *News from a foreign country came*
> *As if my treasure and my heart lay there*

carrying such a wealth of meaning and significance that I could not conceive of any other country worth living in; nor could I understand how its claims could be recon-ciled with any kind of conformity with the rules which govern our ordinary lives.

Yet these rules exist. The time came when at length I had to decide what I was to do with myself, and it was becoming increasingly evident that, short of something totally impossible to foresee, Oxford was the fate or the doom that lay in wait for me. Feebly, spasmodically, I tried to resist. To me it seemed that no life was worth living which did not allow one access to the voices which seemed to speak to me from some invisible sphere, yet even I was not so stupid as to believe that these voices were of a kind to carry me very far on the road to academic success. I forced my father, much against his will, to write to Edward Garnett, with whom he had been friends at the City of London School, to ask his help in placing me as an apprentice to a printer in London, for it seemed to me that in such work one might find the kind of freedom which I wanted and after all, hadn't Blake been a printer? It was with dismay that I read Garnett's very sensible reply that this might mean committing myself to a very hazardous and precarious existence, and that anyone who had any chance of going to Oxford would be very foolish not to make the most of it.

It was not the reply I had hoped for, though indeed I hardly knew myself what I wanted, but short of running away altogether, which for a moment I contemplated, I could see no way of escape. So, reluctantly, I fell in with the wishes of my parents and schoolmasters, and amid my other preoccupations began to study seriously for a scholarship to Oxford. It was also necessary, in order to accumulate sufficient funds, to win a state scholarship, of which at that time there were twelve for the whole of Wales, and awarded strictly by competition on the marks obtained in the Higher School Certificate examination.

I was determined, however, that if I was to sit for a scholarship to Oxford, it should not be in English. It seemed to me that the kind of pleasures I derived from language and from literature could only wither under the dead hand of academic study; what had scholarship to do with the visions and revelations I found in Blake or Donne or Traherne? It seemed to me that literature was far too serious a matter for scholars, who were of necessity divorced from that life of sensation from which literature springs, and I recited to myself Yeat's lines:

> *They'll cough in the ink to the world's end;*
> *Wear out the carpet with their shoes*
> *Earning respect; have no strange friend;*
> *If they have sinned nobody knows.*
> *Lord, what would they say*
> *Should their Catullus walk that way?*

Literature and scholarship seemed to me worlds apart and I could not conceive that the one could be a fit subject for the other. So instead of English I chose history as the subject in which I should specialize; the decision was all the easier because of my respect and admiration for the intellectual standards demanded by my history master. If I could satisfy him, I felt, I could satisfy any examiner; it would also be a delight to study under him, because, himself the son of a village blacksmith in North Wales and a passionate Welshman, he was also a man of unusually wide and varied culture and the least provincial or parochial of men in his vision of what the study of history entailed.

And so indeed it proved. For my last two years at school I followed the course he plotted for me, which included, in addition to English history, the history of medieval Europe and of the French Revolution. Under his tuition, I found history as absorbing and enthralling as anything to be found in literature, and indeed they seemed to be only two different ways of apprehending a single reality; for what was it, after all, to study history but to plunge into that great ocean of the past which laps us round at every moment of our waking and dreaming lives? Or so at least it seemed to me at that time, and I delighted to try and discover in the saints and mystics of the Middle Ages, and in the cathedrals which are their greatest creations, the same vision of reality which I found in poets and artists. The cathedrals indeed seemed to me like vast epics written in stone, great forests of images and dreams drawn from the most secret and sacred recesses of the human heart, through the tracery of whose interlacing branches one caught glimpses of the same heaven and the same hell which are the provinces of all art. And when I passed from the middle ages to the French revolution, how else could I think of Danton bellowing his courage and his despair in his gigantic bull's voice except as yet another of those titanic figures out of *Spiritus Mundi*, as heroic as Achilles or Cuchulain, and perhaps even more because the powers and forces with which he wrestled, like Jacob with the angels, were so much closer to those with which men wrestle in our own time?

I have no doubt there was much that was merely fanciful in my attitude to history and the ideas and images which I imported into it. Now, I cannot help thinking that they tended to bemuse and bewilder me rather than to throw any light on the subject. I do not think that a boy who tries to interpret history according to a system of correspondences borrowed from Baudelaire or a belief in the literal truth of Blake's prophetic books is ever likely to achieve a high degree of objective truth, and I do not think that I ever came very near to understanding the past *wie es eigentlich gewesen war*—as it actually existed. But I do know that the curious, even absurd, hotchpotch of ideas by which I tried to decode the past made of it to me something which was genuinely my own, and of use and value to me in my own life, a living and not a dead thing, which was shot through and through with my own dreams and imaginings; and this at least had the advantage of making the past so fascinating that by the way and almost by accident I absorbed a good deal of knowledge, for even I could not make bricks without any straw at all. When many years later I read Nietzsche's essay *Vom Nützen und Nachteil der Historie für das Leben (Of the Uses and Disadvantages of History in Life)*, I felt grateful that for a time at least it had been the usefulness, in Nietzsche's sense, of history which had been most apparent to me; and perhaps that is an experience which once gained can never be wholly lost. But today I cannot help wondering what kind of stuff it was that, writing in feverish haste and with hardly a pause for thought, I poured out in my examination papers at Oxford and can only wonder at the ability of my examiners to make head or tail of it.

During my last year at school I worked extremely hard, especially in the long winter evenings when I sat bent over my books at the table in our parlour while my mother and father read in silence in their armchairs on either side of the fireplace. The crimson tablecloth on which my books were piled, the glowing light of the fire, fed by the best Welsh coal, the dark mahogany furniture and the Victorian prints on the walls, the scratching of my pen on the paper, the absolute and unbroken silence, induced in me a feeling that time had come to a stop and that we three were preserved for ever in an immobility which change could never threaten. And I was happy that it should be so, for the quiet room with its shadows in the corner where the lamplight never penetrated was transformed into a kind of enchanted cave peopled by all the spirits called up from the past by my books, which I read as if they were works of necromancy that could endow me with magical powers. If I paused for a moment and looked up from my reading, the sense of being encapsuled in some timeless moment, of total and absolute insulation against everything that existed outside those four walls, was so intense that I seemed to float free of my body and to look down on the room as if it were one of those Dutch interiors in which every worn and familiar object, and the faces of those who sit among them, are illuminated by an internal light, a warmth, a glow, a splendour that came from some world which is beyond the world of change.

This was in winter. In summer I worked alone in my bedroom and on golden evenings before the sun had finally set would allow myself the pleasure of walking through the gardens of the public park nearby to hire a

boat and row for an hour on the shallow waters of its
artificial lake. The park would be crowded with the
citizens of Cardiff taking the evening air, trades people
and their wives, courting couples, children bouncing
balls and trundling hoops on the concrete paths between
the symmetrically ordered flower beds, and the presence
of so many others in a world which for me had become
intensely solitary, the contrast with the dreams that filled
my mind, momentarily bewildered and confused me, and
yet this world of flesh and blood was as mysterious and
alluring as anything the imagination had to offer. One
evening I had been reading the *Lyrical Ballads*, and it
seemed to me that it did not need the genius of a Words-
worth to infuse the light of poetry into the sober and
somewhat drab reality of our municipal park, for it was
not a light which we imagined or contrived for ourselves,
as by some trick of stage production, but was as much a
part of these men and women, these trees and flowers,
these stretches of freshly watered grass in the yellowing
evening sunshine as it had been of Adam and Eve as they
walked in the garden of Eden.

The lake stretched beyond the gardens, and in the cool
and mysterious shadows of the trees on the two small
islands at its further end I let the boat float among the
ducks that dabbled in its waters. One section of the lake
was enclosed to form a bathing pool, where on warm
evenings I used to swim and watch the slender long-
legged bodies of the girls who swooped like swallows
from the diving board and flashed like fish through the
waters. To me they seemed like creatures out of mythology,
nymphs, naiads, ondines, water sprites, and when sometimes I summoned up my courage to make their acquaintance I was tongue-tied with shyness and embarrassment
and could find no words to express the confused desire

c

which consumed me. I envied the boldness and brash confidence of my schoolfellows who, when darkness began to fall, would accompany the girls up the hill to the woods above the lake and next day regale the form with boasts of their sexual achievements. Only rarely did I overcome my shyness sufficiently to emulate their example, and then, lying in the grass beside a girl whose dark hair still wet from bathing hung down her back like a mermaid's, made clumsy attempts at love-making which only her more experienced hands, limbs, body, guided to success. But the memory of those girlish bodies—limbs that entwined one like seaweed, the smell as of fresh milk that exuded from their skin—haunted my dreams and blurred my vision as I sat bent over my books and they also had to be included in my vision of the world, in which almost everything else had been derived from literature and not from life.

VII

At length, in the Christmas vacation of 1927, the day arrived when I travelled up to Oxford to take the scholarship examination. I had only once passed beyond the borders of Wales, on a Saturday afternoon coach trip to play football against the Crypt School at Gloucester, and when we passed through the Severn Tunnel it was truly a foreign country that I entered. It was something of a comfort that I was not alone on this voyage of discovery. My companion was a school friend who had the advantage of being a superlative football player, and was therefore assured of some sort of scholarship at Brasenose, which in those days was more like an athletic association than a seat of learning. I had no such advantage and my chances of success at New College were decidedly slimmer. Indeed, they seemed to me non-existent when, after three days of writing examination papers in New College Hall,

I waited in the Warden's lodgings with the other candidates until my turn came to be interviewed.

They seemed to me, as in fact they really were, of another race from myself, or indeed from anyone else I had ever known. Their voices were different, their clothes were different, their manners were different, and to me they even seemed to look different. They all came from public schools, and some of them had been at school together; they had brothers, cousins, friends already at the university, they knew each other's sisters, and for them Oxford was simply the natural and inevitable sequel to school and not the realization of an impossible ambition. They were in no way awestruck or abashed, as I was, by the Gothic ambience of the long gallery in which we waited outside the warden's study. They felt at ease and at home there, and as they waited they lounged gracefully around and gossiped to each other in a manner which seemed to me the height of elegance and sophistication. It struck me forcibly at that moment that they were made for Oxford, in a way which I was not, and Oxford was made for them, and I could see no reason why Oxford, or New College, should go so far out of their normal course as to bestow a scholarship on me, especially as I was still not quite sure whether I wanted one. But though I was not sure what I wanted, I was also combative and competitive and did not at all like the idea that, with all their advantages, these people seemed certain to succeed where I seemed equally bound to fail.

It was not that I thought them cleverer, or more intelligent, or better educated than myself. Some hidden source of self-confidence or vanity told me that they were not. It was simply that in the long medieval gallery, with the portraits of past wardens hanging on the wall, they moved as naturally as fish in water while I hardly dared to speak for fear of attracting attention to my uncouthness, to my Welsh voice, to my ill-fitting suit, my lack of any of the social accomplishments which sat so easily on them. It was really all quite simple; they were at home and I was not.

I felt strangely naked and vulnerable when I entered the Warden's study and found the Warden and some of the Fellows seated in a semi-circle which I faced from a chair beside the fire. What comforted me, though it came almost as a shock because I had entirely failed to foresee it, was the tone of kindness and friendliness in which all their questions were directed at me, the politeness of the interest with which they listened to my answers, the air of ease and urbanity, of gentle consideration, with which the interview was conducted, and in those few moments the seeds of an abiding affection for Oxford were implanted in my heart. It was less like an interview than a form of seduction.

There was a charm in it which conquered me, so that when at length the interview was over and I made my way home from New College to my room in St Aldate's, for the first time I felt a real regret that perhaps I might never see Oxford again. I had felt, for a moment, a sense that Oxford might have much to teach me, in matters not only of learning but of living. When I left the next morning to stay for the weekend in London with my grandmother, I felt that if I had failed I should be the loser in more senses than one. So that when on the following day I received a telegram informing me that I had been awarded an open scholarship, I was not only gratified by the sense of having achieved something that was not easy. I felt also, with a certain stirring of excitement, that I was on the verge of making new discoveries and that, whether I wished it or not, a new and different world was opening out before me.

Two

My childhood and youth, and the slightly odd person they had made of me, were perhaps not the best sort of preparation for Oxford as it was when I first proceeded there at the age of eighteen in the autumn of 1928. For in those days Oxford was still very much of a closed society, with its own traditions, even its own morality, all of which were as strange and alien to me as if I had suddenly found myself in Timbuctoo or Kamchatka.

This is not to say that Oxford at that time was a completely homogeneous and monolithic society, with which I alone was out of step. Like all societies, it had its own internal divisions and distinctions into the interstices of which a stranger might settle himself with a reasonable amount of comfort. They were not, as they were to become later, political divisions, because politics had not yet assumed that dominating part in the life of the university which it was to play in the thirties. Nor was there the slightest sign, at that time, of the general revolt of the young against the old, of the taught against the teacher, which has become a characteristic feature of the universities today. In this respect, both dons and undergraduates lived in a kind of age of innocence, in which neither had as yet discovered that they hated each other.

Undergraduates indeed were, by modern standards of student revolt, a singularly amenable and submissive lot. This was largely due to the fact that for most of them Oxford presented a blissful liberation from the restrictions imposed on them at their public schools. If the yoke of the university, and of the colleges, would seem intolerably heavy to the undergraduate of today, it was then easily borne because it was so much lighter than what had gone before. Youthful revolt was directed, not against the university, but against the public school system; quite a large library could have been collected of adolescent novels in which, from *The Loom of Youth* onwards, their authors described the tortures and sufferings imposed on them at school, as if they had escaped from some premature form of concentration or labour camp. To read them, one would have thought that the entire middle class had in its youth been the victim of an organized system of educational terrorism. The scars, however, had not penetrated very deep, and in no way prevented the victims, while licking their wounds, from enjoying the liberties and pleasures they were now offered; rather, they only added a keener and sharper flavour to them.

Politics, in the form in which they have manifested themselves both in the 1930s and the 1960s, have so transformed the Oxford which I first knew that today I hardly find it recognizable. The greatest change they have introduced is the assumption that the university is no longer a preparation for adult life, an interlude in which the undergraduate, half boy, half man, is not yet fully grown, but is already a part of the adult world, with the same intensely practical concerns and interests, among which is the inescapable duty of changing it for the better.

In this sense, it could be said that Oxford, in 1928, was still in the pre-industrial stage of its history, enjoying the last golden glow of a kind of pastoral civilization which had endured, in some respects unchanged, since the Middle Ages; this was true even of its physical environment, because the name of Morris did not yet fully spell out the doom which the internal combustion engine would bring upon the city and the university. Perhaps this lack of adaptation was Oxford's condemnation; but it did not make it any the less enjoyable. Of course, even then, there were little enclaves in the university in which politics reared their ugly head. There was, for instance, the Oxford Union, a kind of school debating society for budding professional politicians, but no one except a very small minority of its members took its proceedings very seriously, and certainly no one would have dreamed of attributing to them the kind of importance they assumed when, only a few years later, the Union with typical frivolity carried its famous resolution "That this house will not fight for King and Country". And there was already at Oxford, and particularly at New College, a group of admirably serious and dedicated young men who many years later, after many vicissitudes, would provide the Labour party with an entirely new leadership and stamp it with their own peculiar form of Wykehamist socialism.

But they also were exceptional, both in their intelligence and the seriousness with which they prepared themselves for the life of politics. They already exuded an air of professionalism and puritanism which was somehow out-of-tune with the fin-de-siècle atmosphere of the end of the twenties. It was perhaps a sign of my own frivolity that, though I thought of myself as a socialist, I found their ideas altogether too humdrum and dreary to fit into my Utopian dreams of revolution. Equally, perhaps, there was something in their public-school version of socialism which offended against instincts which were rooted in my origins. Somehow it was tainted by the charitable, and estimable, motive of "doing something for the poor". I felt that I was one of the poor myself, and was not at all sure I wanted them to do something for me.

Politics was not yet a cause of contention. Nor was age. The university was still by modern standards very small and a college was hardly more than a large family. Married dons were the exception and not the rule, their strictly academic duties relatively very light and there were few distractions to turn their minds away from Oxford. Dons and undergraduates lived in an intimacy which is no longer possible and by knowing each other overcame the barriers of age and learned a mutual affection which today has largely disappeared from university life.

The most obvious division within the university when I first arrived there was between the Hearties and the Aesthetes. The Hearty saw himself as representing virility as opposed to decadence, the Aesthete was the selfconscious champion of culture against barbarism. Hearties went in for beer and games, club scarves and blazers, fast cars and motor cycles, picking up girls on Saturday night in the Carfax assembly rooms, and throwing Quintin Hogg into Mercury, the pool that adorns Tom Quad at Christchurch. Aesthetes were dedicated to poetry and the arts, they were, or affected to be, homosexual, spent their holidays in Germany and came back with stories of the wonderful decadence of the Weimar Republic; in dress and appearance they reflected, at long range and modified to suit English tastes, the image of the dandy created by Baudelaire. Hearties and Aesthetes alike boasted representative types who displayed the characteristic features of the species in their most extreme form; on the one hand the oafish rowing man whose greatest pleasure was the wrecking of some studious and inoffensive undergraduate's rooms after a bump supper, on the other some exotic immigrant like the Queen of Peru, a South American male tart who, amid surroundings of Second Empire Parisian splendour, held court in rooms somewhere off Beaumont Street.

Between these two camps there raged an undeclared war; they represented as it were the two poles towards which undergraduate life gravitated. They were divided by a kind of plain or marsh, neutral ground in which the majority of undergraduates had their being, uncommitted to either side but each responding in his particular way to the pull exerted by the one or the other. There were poets who, though by every other sign they were to be recognized as Aesthetes, were as devoted to beer and football as any Hearty; there were athletes who, off the track or river, were as intellectual in their tastes as any aesthete. And there were many who simply took the pleasures Oxford had to offer as they came, without bothering too much about what they implied, content, and more than content, to spend their three years there as if they formed one long summer afternoon.

In this no-man's-land which was the abode of the average undergraduate, I managed to create a particular limbo of my own. Inclination and temperament led me towards the aesthetes, whose taste for literature and the arts I shared; but at the same time I remained fond, as I had been at school, of playing games and this made me something of an eccentric in their ranks.

But if, in the company of friends, I often had the sense of being not wholly accepted, or acceptable, I felt it even more strongly with regard to Oxford life in general. For the divisions and distinctions within the university, of which that between the Hearty and the Aesthete was only the most obvious, were only superficial as compared with the social uniformity which Oxford presented to a stranger like myself. For Oxford was then still an almost exclusive monopoly of what Keynes somewhere calls "the great capitalist class" and its breeding ground, the public schools. Interlopers from the state educational system formed so small a minority that we made scarcely any impression upon the system as a whole, which could afford to tolerate, even welcome, our presence because we represented no kind of threat to its cohesiveness. New College, particularly, represented a special case of this general condition. It owed its existence to the same founder as Winchester College, William of Wykeham, and an unbroken historical connection between the two institutions, together with a generous provision of closed scholarships, made it a special preserve of Wykehamists. They gave the college a particular sub-culture of its own, and an historian of manners would have been fascinated to observe how precisely they conformed, after so many centuries, though in modern dress as it were, to the pattern of piety, respect for scholarship, and dedication to the service of Church and State, which had been the idea of the founder.

Of such sub-cultures there was an almost bewildering variety at Oxford, flourishing not only in particular colleges but in every kind of undergraduate club, association and society, and, even more perhaps, in purely ephemeral and transitory groups of friends bound together by nothing more than common tastes and interests, which might vary from bird-watching to seventeenth-century music. It was for me one of the particular charms of the place that one might stumble across such mini-cultures in the most unlikely corners. I used to sally out from my rooms in New College like a traveller following the course of an unexplored river, never knowing what strange flora and fauna, what exotic tribes and customs, one might encounter on its banks.

One of the oddest, perhaps, of such societies, which I came across rather late in my university life, was a group of three undergraduates who shared rooms together far off in Wellington Square. They rarely ventured out except to attend lectures and tutorials, and their rooms themselves had the grim and cheerless austerity of a monastic cell. No pictures adorned their walls, and their bookshelves displayed only a few works of the most rigorous scholarship; the very air in them seemed to breathe abstraction. There they shared together a life devoted entirely to a peculiarly refined and rigorous process of self-examination, like medieval flagellants chastising themselves and each other with the whips of logical analysis. No intellectual peccadillo was so trivial that it escaped each other's condemnation; no social distraction so innocent that it did not provoke a frown of disapproval, almost of disgust; no sign of frivolity, intellectual or moral, that did not represent a fall from grace. Their only concession to self-indulgence was, so far as I knew, a cup of cocoa at bedtime as they listened to a Bach concerto. When, fascinated by the penances they imposed on each other, I used to visit them, I used to be greeted with a chilly and disapproving silence, and felt like some butterfly which has violated the privacy of an anchorite's cell; but the strangest thing about it all was that they were, all three of them, blissfully happy.

At a different extreme, there were those for whom Oxford provided an opportunity for almost total idleness and dissipation, though even these sometimes assumed eccentric forms. A friend whom I had not known as an undergraduate later confessed to me that his life at Oxford had followed a rigidly determined pattern, which never varied from day to day. At eleven o'clock in the morning he was woken by his scout with an orange and a glass of brandy, which formed his breakfast. He then shaved, bathed and dressed, and strolled to the Carlton Club where he lunched, each day, on a grilled steak and a bottle of claret. The afternoon was spent in a cinema, and from five to six he played billiards with the professional at the university billiards club. Returning to college, he made ready for the evening, which was spent in dining with friends and consuming large quantities of alcohol. By twelve he was back in college, and retired to bed; and at eleven the following morning his scout appeared with an orange and a glass of brandy, and the daily routine was repeated. After two years he felt that he had learned everything Oxford had to teach him and, without regret and without a degree, left the university to prepare for the serious business of life by going to work in a factory in Birmingham. This case history of idleness, however, concealed a talent which later made its subject a very distinguished novelist, Henry Green.

Not many undergraduates, of course, devised quite so bizarre a programme for spending their time at Oxford, though I have no doubt that if one looked into the darker corners of some of the more obscure colleges one would have found recluses who were enjoying themselves in an equally eccentric fashion. Indeed it was precisely the charm of Oxford at that time that, within the not very demanding limits of college and university discipline, it allowed young men to spend their time exactly as they pleased, with the least possible interference of any kind of authority, and encouraged them to indulge their tastes, whether frivolous or serious, with a liberty which few societies have ever permitted their members.

There is a story of the great German classical scholar, Williamowitz-Möllendorf, that once, on a visit to Oxford, he was taken to the top of Magdalen Tower on a summer's afternoon and from there looked down at the streets and buildings spread out beneath him. The town was still then much as Gerard Manley Hopkins described it in *Duns Scotus's Oxford:*

> *Towery city and branchy between towers*
> *Cuckoo-echoing, bell-swarmèd, lark-charmèd,*
> *rook-racked, river rounded;*

and on an afternoon in May its streets were filled with undergraduates in white flannels or rowing kit making their way to the river or the cricket field or the tennis court. And the great scholar averted his eyes from the scene and scornfully spat out the words: *Eine Luststadt!* (A pleasure resort!)

A pleasure resort! It certainly was to me; yet I do not know that, in the end, the grim austerities of Prussian scholarship have served the cause of learning, or of civilization, better than the more humane traditions of Oxford. I have no doubt that, in my own time, there were people who were as committed to the most exacting forms of scholarship, and spent their days, and their nights, as laboriously as even Williamowitz could have wished. But even in them it was love not duty or discipline which drove them to their labours, and the harsh demands of scholarship were sweetened and mellowed by Oxford's air of freedom and toleration, by acceptance of the Rabelaisian doctrine of *Do What Thou Wilt is the Whole of the Law*; most of all perhaps by acceptance of Mark Pattison's belief that the final end and object of scholarship is not a book, but a man.

As for the rest of us, learning, if it was of any interest, was only one among the many other pleasures Oxford had to offer. Some managed to get on very happily without any learning at all. I myself did not totally succumb to Oxford's particularly seductive form of hedonism; but if there was anything which I took away with me from Oxford it was the belief that learning is a kind of pleasure and pleasure a kind of learning, even if it is only the pleasure of learning about oneself. On the whole it is a belief which is conducive to happiness, though perhaps it is not a very good guide to the sterner realities of life. But it always seemed then that there would be plenty of time for them later.

In this respect Oxford, when I first arrived there, was not perhaps the best of preparations for a future which was to turn out far uglier than anyone might have reasonably expected. It was still bathed in a kind of golden glow, as of a setting sun, which allowed a certain class of young Englishman a kind of happiness which I do not think has been possible for him since. For the end of the twenties was perhaps the last time the English ruling classes, and their children who were my contemporaries and friends, could look forward with any confidence to the continuation of the kind of world on which their privileges and their prosperity depended. That confidence had already been severely shaken by the First World War and its immediate aftermath in Europe of revolution, the fall of dynasties, the collapse of ancient empires; the wisest perhaps already knew that there could be no real recovery from so great a disaster, but if so this was a wisdom which was reserved only for the few. Since 1924 the world had enjoyed an unprecedented economic boom, and stable political conditions had been re-established; and Britain also had shared in the general restoration of confidence which this inspired, the revival of hope, the sense that after all total disaster had been averted and that the world could look forward to a new era of peace and prosperity in which Britain would still play a dominant if slightly diminished part.

It seemed as if the lights which had been extinguished

in 1914 had gone up again. Europe, which Herman Hesse had seen in 1920 as "on the way to chaos, staggering drunkenly in holy madness on the edge of the abyss, singing like Dimitri Karamazov in drunkenness and ecstasy", had been restored to financial and political stability. The United States was enjoying an economic boom so prodigious that every country in the world felt its effects. The Covenant of the League of Nations and the Pact of Locarno guaranteed the world, and particularly Europe, against a renewal of the aggressive and bellicose policies which had provoked the tragedy of 1914. In such conditions, even the Kellogg–Briand Pact outlawing war in perpetuity did not read like a fairy story, and the preparations for the World Disarmament Conference seemed to promise that the entire world would beat its swords into ploughshares; was not even Krupp doing so already at Essen?

No doubt the happy expectations inspired by so astonishing a recovery from the depths of disaster were largely based on illusion, but in 1928 it would have taken a wise man to realize it, and undergraduates are not, on the whole, very wise, nor were their teachers any wiser. Their fathers' recovery of assurance and confidence, the general feeling that all Britain now needed was a policy of enlightened apathy, was reflected in the sons by a sense that the world was their oyster, and the only difficulty was what particular breed of oyster to select. Some chose learning, some chose art, some chose self-indulgence, some chose games; some even chose rebellion against their fathers and everything they represented, but with a subconscious assurance that this also was only another kind of game and nothing very serious would happen as a result. And whatever the choice there was an underlying assumption that what mattered was to choose for oneself, and that the sum of individual choices could only contribute to the greatest happiness of all.

Of course, for the undergraduate, there were limitations to the liberty which he enjoyed, but they were easy to bear because they were the price of his privileges. In this respect Oxford was more like a club than a modern university, and despite the still almost medieval domestic arrangements of the colleges, the undergraduate lived in considerable comfort, which in some respects at least amounted to luxury. With his own bedroom and sitting room, which at any moment could be totally sealed off from the outside world by the simple expedient of "sporting his oak", he enjoyed an enviable degree of privacy. The services of his scout relieved him of all domestic cares and responsibilities. The precise degree of luxury with which he surrounded himself was a function of his, or rather his father's, income; if it were large enough, he could afford to indulge every taste, from lavish hospitality to keeping polo ponies. But the basic luxury was the independence and privacy which every undergraduate enjoyed, the sense of being able to live and breathe in a space of his own and of freedom from interference with what he chose to do with his own time. There was, of course, the risk of being sent down if he wasted it too conspicuously; but this, after all, was very much a matter of his own choice.

To me at least these were luxuries indeed. By the standards of most of my contemporaries I was poor, but a state scholarship, a college scholarship, and a scholarship from the city of Cardiff provided me with a total income of £250 a year, which to me was wealth. It was sufficient to cover my basic needs, largely supplied by the college, and enabled me to buy as many books as I wanted, clothe myself, and indulge in whatever minor pleasures, though none of the major extravagances, that I chose. There was even the special pleasure of never needing to have any money in one's pocket, for cash was quite unnecessary when everything was to be had on credit. My own debts, after three years at Oxford, amounted to £70, which were promptly paid for by my father, without question, reproach or hesitation.

Thus, on arrival at Oxford, I suddenly enjoyed the illusion of total financial independence and for me this was one of the uncovenanted graces of being an undergraduate. It was an illusion which, once acquired, I never wholly lost, even when any justification for it had disappeared, and in later life this led me into many mistakes. For of course we never really are independent, whatever we may think or feel, and perhaps it is best if we come to realize this at an early age. But this was a thought which, if it had occurred to me, I should certainly have rejected with scorn and contempt. My newly acquired freedom seemed to me absolute and the only urgent problem, if one could call it such, was what one was going to do with it.

Such an attitude seems all the more curious to me now because I believed myself to be a socialist and a Marxist, a worshipper at the shrine of what was sometimes familiarly referred to as the MCH; the Materialist Conception of History. For me this was an important article of faith; but somehow I felt that, though it applied to everyone else, it did not apply to me. This, however, was only one of the many contradictions which I had no difficulty in accepting at that time. After all, were not contradictions an essential part of the dialectic?

Perhaps it was the inscrutable working of the dialectic, or merely something contrary in my own nature which ensured that, though aware of my own good fortune, I was more often than not miserable at Oxford. I was lonely, and felt the need of my parents and home. I missed the intimate, fire-lit domesticity of our sitting room at night, the silence which reigned when we sat together in the long winter evenings; I missed the city streets and the girls in the park and the feeling that, even when one was alone, the city and its people and the dark valleys groping like outstretched fingers into the coalfield, were packed close around one, dense, mysterious, yet familiar. For in Oxford I was a stranger, and remained one. The city played no part in one's life; girls rarely penetrated it; my rooms, high up in Gilbert Scott's New Buildings, or, later, in the garden quadrangle, seemed bare and austere compared with home, and the El Greco reproductions I had hung on their walls sometimes seemed to throw a lurid and sinister glare on their emptiness.

Dining in Hall, under the high oak roof that multiplied the din of the dinner tables, I would listen to the conversation around me, and the English middle-class voices sometimes seemed to be the voices of foreigners, speaking an alien tongue; or rather it was I who was the alien, surrounded by people of whose manners and customs I knew nothing. For it was not only differences of language, voice, accent, which divided us; tricks of phrase and turns of speech revealed the gulf between two nations and two cultures.

"Do you know the Angleseys?" an aristocratic and very beautiful young man said to me one evening as we were drinking sherry in the buttery; sherry was the staple drink of the day and sometimes we seemed to drown in butts of it, like the Duke of Clarence in malmsey.

"The Angleseys?" I said. "There's only one of them." He was as puzzled by my reply as I was by his question, and it was some time before I learned that the name of a

72

place could also be the name of a person or a family. And when I did, it was with something of the same sense of poetic discovery with which Proust learned that names which for him conveyed the blood-shot mysteries of the Dark Ages were also the titles of living people. The Angleseys, I felt, must have all the gentle charm and beauty, the legendary fertility, as of heaped-up corn, of the island from which they took their name.

Such misunderstandings showed what a rich and varied field of exploration Oxford offered, and after a time they were enough to tempt me out of my nineteenth-century Gothic tower in New College. There was of course more familiar ground for me to frequent. I could, for instance, have sought the company of compatriots, including some of my schoolfellows, who were at Oxford at that time. They were mostly concentrated in Jesus, *Coleg yr Jesu*, a kind of Patagonian colony in the Turl, where they cultivated the Welsh language and the nostalgia which the Welsh call *Hiraeth*, and in general lived the life of exiles for whom Oxford was only a form of foreign posting before they returned again to their native land. But I had no wish to join this kind of Welsh old-colonial society. If Oxford were to be of any value at all, I felt, it would only be if it offered a wider and more varied world than Wales. Otherwise I might just as well, perhaps better, have stayed at home. What was the point of the pains of parting if they brought me nothing new?

Fortunately, curiosity alone was enough to drive me abroad, and gradually I began to make friends, at first in my own college, and later elsewhere, both with undergraduates and with dons, who in those days were willing to devote what now seems an almost inordinate amount of their time and their affection to undergraduates. To me, these new friendships had something of the pleasure

73

and excitement of foreign travel; I felt as if I were conducting a kind of miniature Grand Tour of English society, as reflected in the microcosm of Oxford. But sometimes, equally, I saw myself as a spy, dispatched on some desperate mission abroad, whose success depended above all on disguising his identity by a process of protective colouration and on the thoroughness with which he adopted the manners and customs of the country to which he had been assigned.

In such a rôle, I was to some extent protected against such exposure, because I was at that time extremely, perhaps, for my own good, excessively impressionable, quick to adopt all the imitative devices which are necessary for survival in an alien environment, and equally quick to discard anything which might reveal how little I was at home in it. I exploited such gifts, or faults, to the full, so that much of my time was spent in an elaborate exercise in simulation. I do not know how successful it was, and I dare say that it was a good deal less successful than I imagined. But there was a certain pleasure in the performance, even though it imposed a considerable strain, which revealed itself in frequent attacks of the depression which has afflicted me all my life and made me often a difficult companion, most of all to myself.

Such a temperament provided a very precarious basis for my social life at Oxford, which became increasingly a matter of friendships, of parties, of drinking rather more than was good for me, of "nights spent in arguments and ignorant good will" and of generally neglecting my work. Fortunately, terms at Oxford were admirably short, so that it was never necessary to maintain any disguise for more than eight weeks. When they were over, and the vacation came, I could return home, as to a refuge where no disguises were necessary. This happy arrangement also helped to solve the problem of how to combine my exploration of English life, as represented by Oxford, with the necessary amount of work required to satisfy the demands of the curriculum. My scholarships were quite sufficient to cover my needs during term but left little over for the vacations; they were periods of financial stringency in which I made up for the extravagances of term by strict economy at home. Thus gradually term came to represent to me the season of pleasure, the vacation a period of penance in which I laboured to make up for my idleness at Oxford. It was a curious reversal of the academic calendar, but on the whole the arrangement worked very well. Perhaps it explains why my memories of Oxford are coloured with the idea of frivolity and self-indulgence; the world's work, and mine, took place elsewhere.

During term I hardly worked at all, apart from producing a weekly essay for my tutor, and never succeeded in completing a single course of lectures, partly because most of them did not seem to be worth attending, partly because I learned better and faster from books; but mostly because regular attendance would have seriously interfered with my other preoccupations. I made friends, and these were the greatest benefit Oxford conferred on me. I read a great deal, but this was a confirmed addiction before I ever arrived at Oxford. I discovered Proust, who became an obsession to me, and I tended to view my own flibbertigibbet existence through his spectacles and to see in my acquaintances a Baron de Charlus, a Bloch, a Cottard. I also learned some German and acquired a taste for German literature which has remained with me through life, long after Germany had ceased to be fashionable and at times when Germany herself seemed to deny all the values on which her literature is founded.

Despite bouts of depression I enjoyed myself excessively, so that my undergraduate days have retained in memory a special colour and a special flavour, as if drenched in some special ichor that was only distilled at that time and at that place.

But all this, alas! had nothing to do with my academic work. In my first year I had changed my school from History to Modern Greats, in the mistaken belief that philosophy, politics and economics provided the key to the secrets of real life, but they were singularly reluctant to yield them up to me. My new studies never acquired for me the charm which history had once had and I was delighted when, walking in Christchurch meadow, a friend, A. J. Ayer, triumphantly announced to me that he had solved all the problems of philosophy which would shortly, therefore, become a dead subject. But to me it only remained a difficult and intractable one, and distaste only accentuated my idleness. It became sufficiently noticeable to provoke warnings from my tutors and even from my friends that unless I mended my ways I was unlikely to obtain the kind of degree expected or hoped of me as a scholar of the college. The college chaplain, a distinguished theologian to whom my father had commended me, was particularly distressed. "He is *far* too great a social success!" he wailed, in his high nasal voice that always sounded as if he were intoning the lesson in chapel; "he will *never* get a First!" I think his distress was increased because he regarded me as in some sense in his pastoral care. In my third year we lived on the same staircase in the garden quad and he was continually finding pretexts for entering my rooms. Starting out of my chair from a drunken slumber on a winter's afternoon, I found his slightly simian countenance bent over me, his hands on my biceps as he shook me out of sleep.

"You must be eee-mensely strong!" he intoned as I struggled to my feet.

By contrast with such absurd scenes, home and vacations came to represent long hours of study, by which one paid for what one had enjoyed. My friends went away on glamorous foreign travels, to Germany, to France, to Italy; I remained, somewhat enviously, at home, to settle down once again at the sitting-room table, where on the maroon tablecloth medieval saints and mystics had been replaced by Locke and Berkeley and Hume and Kant, with whom I wrestled in growing dismay as I realized that I had no talent for philosophy. And this division, not of labour, but between labour at home and pleasure at Oxford, accentuated for me the sense of living a double life. However much one enjoyed being at Oxford, one never felt that one properly belonged there and would always remain in some sense an interloper; while at home, labouring at neglected studies, one always felt that there was a part of me, idle and pleasure-loving, which had been left behind at Oxford, a frivolous ghost haunting the garden at New College, waiting for the beginning of term to be brought back to life again. It was not altogether an unpleasant feeling.

II

The first invitation I received at Oxford was to play bridge with a Wykehamist scholar who lived on the next staircase to me in New College. I had no business to accept the invitation, as I hardly knew how to play bridge; also I guessed that I should have to play for money, and had visions of incurring losses beyond my means. Both my fears proved correct. Nevertheless I accepted; I had spent nearly every evening alone since my arrival at Oxford, and it had begun to seem to me that my stay there was to be spent in a kind of solitary confinement.

The three undergraduates with whom I played bridge that evening became my firm friends during my three years at New College, and I spent many similar evenings playing bridge with them. I never became a good bridge player and I always lost more money than I could afford, but I do not regard those evenings as wasted, because they afforded an opportunity of observing the English character at its most typical and characteristic. Indeed, my three bridge-playing friends were in many ways so typical of the class from which Oxford was then almost exclusively recruited, that perhaps I could not describe it better than in terms of my meetings with them on that first, and on many subsequent occasions.

Bridge is a game that very quickly exposes a player's temperamental virtues and vices and my three companions that first evening were no different in this respect than any other three card players chosen at random. These three, however, were not chosen at random, for they were all three the carefully selected products of a social system which bred to type as truly and carefully as any scientifically managed racing stud. This is not to say that it suppressed individual variations. Rather, they were encouraged, but only so long as they did not interfere with the preservation of the species. But by some mysterious social process, akin to the bio-chemistry of genetic inheritance, individual variations were so modified and transmuted that in the end it was the characteristics not of the individual but of the type that were dominant.

My three companions were all scholars of the college, and all came from the very best public schools. I do not know what motive had encouraged that first invitation. Perhaps it was curiosity, as in some curious breed of animal they had never previously encountered; or perhaps they had simply taken pity on my isolation, because there was a genuine kindness in their welcome, which, however, took the form of taking it for granted that we were all exactly like each other. Very early in the evening, I realized that they had so much in common in the way of social background, education, mutual friends and shared experiences that they were able to talk in a kind of conversational shorthand, in which a large part of their meaning was unspoken and suppressed; they were like the tips of three icebergs projecting from a vast ocean in which the greater part of them was submerged. Later, I learned to recognize this as a characteristic of a certain class of Englishman, who, because he plays, or played, a dominant part in English society, is often taken by the foreigner to be the type of the Englishman as such and judged alternatively to be mysterious, rude or arrogant. Yet it is not mystery, or rudeness or arrogance which dictates his behaviour; it is a rather topsy-turvy kind of politeness, which assumes that whatever is known to themselves is known equally to all and has no need of explanation.

Indeed to me the conversation that evening was, by reason of the density of its implications and unspoken assumptions, almost unintelligible. A large part of it centred on comparisons of their experiences at school; my knowledge of public-school life was confined to the novels of Talbot Baines Reed and the adventures of Billy Bunter, but Greyfriars seemed to provide no kind of model by which to judge their gossip about Winchester or Eton.

Equally mysterious, and disconcerting to me, was the assurance and confidence with which they faced the present and the future; the element of chance, of the unexpected, seemed to have been eliminated from both. One intended to enter the Civil Service, and preferably the Treasury, and it did not occur to him or to anyone else that a good classical degree might not be the best possible qualification for such a career. Why should it? For nearly a hundred years it had been taken for granted that the classics provided the best possible preparation for administering the nation's financial affairs and there was no reason for thinking that this would be any less true in the future than in the past.

A second had chosen the Sudan service; the sands of the desert had for him the glamour and romance of empire, and if he had any doubt about the future it was merely whether he would get a blue at hockey, because the colonial service regarded some form of athletic distinction as an advantage in governing coloured peoples. He had not considered the possibility that, within his own lifetime, there might no longer be any Empire to govern. With boyish enthusiasm he saw himself in the Sudan following Gordon and Kitchener across the desert to bring civilization to the Fuzzy-Wuzzies. A third was interested in becoming, by way of the bar, a Conservative politician, and proposed to devote much of his time to the activities of the Oxford Union. As for me, I had not the slightest idea of what I intended to do or be, and indeed it seemed to me very possible that no-one would ever be likely to give me any kind of useful employment. After all, back in Wales there were thousands of better men than I to whom life offered no prospect except the bread line and the dole.

All three of my friends that evening were well-educated, intelligent and able. They had been well-taught at school and what they understood they understood very well; what they did not understand included almost everything which would change the world in their lifetime. They took it for granted that, with a moderate degree of application, the highest offices in the state, the law, administration or business were theirs for the asking, except that business still had something of its old, ugly, connotation of *trade* and was not really a proper occupation for a gentleman. The strange thing was that, so far as they themselves were concerned, their assumptions proved to be correct. Despite economic collapse, wars, revolutions, nothing did in fact happen to them to frustrate their hopes and ambitions, and the careers they proposed for themselves were in fact the careers they successfully followed for most of their lives.

They were, I later realized, a very representative cross-section of John Maynard Keynes's "great capitalist class" which in the nineteenth century had made Britain, and to a large extent the world, what they were, and at that moment it appeared that it would continue to do so for the foreseeable future. It is true that, by birth, temperament and inclination my three bridge-playing friends were conservatives. But in other rooms in New College, or elsewhere in Oxford that night, there were other young men who were socialists, and who shared the unconscious assumption that by some in-built providence which worked in favour of the products of Oxford and Cambridge they too belonged to the governing class; curiously enough, some thirty-five years later they also proved to be right. Political differences between undergraduates might be large, even sometimes violent; but in their underlying belief that the world was theirs for the asking, they were alike as eggs from the same basket.

To me, however, it would have seemed incredible at that time that so bland a certainty about the future would in fact turn out to be justified. The particular version of socialism which I professed was an extremely confused and incoherent one. So far as ideas went it was largely derived from Marx, William Morris and George Bernard Shaw; emotionally it was deeply coloured by a kind of naive industrial populism, based upon an intense admiration for the South Wales miners and an acute sense of what seemed to me the injustices which they suffered in their lives and in their work. If I had been asked what I wanted or hoped for, and if I had answered truthfully, I think I would have said that it was a world governed by the South Wales Miners' Federation. My new friends' expectations from life, based upon the prescriptive right to power and privilege of the class to which they belonged, were an offence to everything I believed, which was roughly that some day soon everything would be made anew and that in this glorious apocalypse I too might find a place amongst those who on the appointed day would arise as if transfigured from the dead. For I had an incurable habit of thinking in images and if anything this grew upon me at Oxford, because as an undergraduate I discovered a love of painting and in particular of the Italian and German primitives which I had been able to see in the Ashmolean and, on my rare visits to London, in the National Gallery. Admiration for Proust had made me read Ruskin, and, after him, Berenson and Burckhardt. Visual images further confused my intellectual processes, if such they could be called. Revolution presented itself to me as in some *quattrocento* vision in the Biblical imagery which I had learned in the chapel, in the shape of men and women who, out of great tribulation, and from the pits and valleys of Wales, had come to History's great seat of judgement. *Die Weltgeschichte ist das Weltgericht!* I could not think that the verdict could now be long postponed nor that it would be given in favour of those who, from Oxford, looked forward so confidently to the future.

Of course, I would not have confessed, even to myself, that my socialism was so coloured by such childishly apocalyptic dreams, as if it were made up out of those coloured lithographs which illustrated the text of our Welsh Bibles. I regarded myself as a strictly rational being, whose political beliefs were based on science and hard fact and might even have formed a proper subject for an essay for my tutor. But in reality they were the product of a part of me I did not understand, and hardly cared to enquire into, and this being so, in argument or debate they left me with feelings of irritation and frustration, as if the real meaning of what I wished to say escaped me, and always would escape me, however hard I might try to put it into words.

No such doubts or frustrations, I think, afflicted my bridge-playing companions and indeed, to the eye of a stranger and newcomer, one of their most striking characteristics was a certain complacency, as if even so early in life they already knew exactly who and what they were and what they would become and saw no reason to be dissatisfied with the knowledge. For me, this conferred an air of mystery on them which was almost certainly a product of my own imagination. I saw them like fishes moving slowly and sedately within a transparent tank, lazily stirring its weeds and grasses with their fins and staring out through its glass walls with eyes that were blind to everything except what went on within. Later, as I came to know them better, I used sometimes to feel a sense of anger that nothing had ever happened, nothing perhaps might ever happen, in spite of all my hopes, to ruffle their assurance; but even at that first meeting I also felt a sense of disappointment because I knew I could never share with them any of the ideas and feelings which had so occupied my mind in my later years at school.

There seemed to be lacking in them some principle of the imagination which was all that I valued at the time, and which somehow I wished to see translated into reality. They had seen a great deal more of the world than I had, and, to judge by their conversation, the future seemed to offer them wider opportunities than were open to me; yet somehow I felt assured that whatever happened to them, however unexpected or surprising it might be, it would lose all of its particular essence by being translated into the forms and categories by which their minds were circumscribed.

This seemed all the more likely because I could see no evidence that their ideas had ever ventured beyond the limits approved by their parents and their schoolmasters. When I had the opportunity to wander round the room and look at its books and pictures and ornaments it was quickly clear that one could not expect to find anything that would not have satisfied the conventional taste of twenty-five years earlier; some Greek and Latin texts, *A Shropshire Lad*, school groups, photographs of Mummy and Daddy. There was nothing to suggest that in the interval there had been a revolution in ideas and in tastes, nor indeed was there any reflection of it in their conversation, which, apart from the formal jargon of the bridge table, consisted chiefly of gossip about people I didn't know, reminiscences of school which I did not understand, and accounts of holidays abroad in places where I had never been.

Yet despite my disappointment, I could not deny to myself that I had found the evening agreeable. It was a relief from loneliness, all the more acceptable because of the genuine friendliness of my new acquaintances' welcome, their general assumption that my being there at all made me of their own kind. If they talked of matters of which I knew nothing, it was not in order to exclude me but because they took it for granted that they were as familiar to me as to themselves. Otherwise, what was I doing at Oxford at all?

I should not have found it at all easy to answer that question myself. It was rather as if I had joined a club without realizing what I was doing. But fortunately the question never seemed to arise because, as time passed, I found myself too preoccupied with the distractions Oxford offered to wonder whether, as far as I was concerned, they served any good purpose. Indeed, the initial disappointment I had suffered did not last. Later, I made friends who shared my own interests, and widened and deepened them, and in this sense at least Oxford did not disappoint me. They varied as widely in temperament and intelligence and character as people do anywhere else; but what gave them, for me, an added fascination was that they also, in all their variety, displayed so clearly the marks of the English ruling class from which they all sprang; indeed, their individual differences seemed only to emphasize its almost infinite ramifications and complications. A youthful, rebellious left-wing poet, at odds with every social and sexual convention, nevertheless did not fail to display, in all his personal dealings, the native shrewdness and powers of calculation of the Jewish banking dynasty from which his money was derived. An embryo musician, who neglected all his studies to devote himself to Schönberg and Webern, and to passionate homosexual affairs, still had about him the faintly clerical air of the cathedral close in which his parents and grandparents had lived. Indeed the extravagances, personal and intellectual, in which so many of my friends indulged were in some respects simply a kind of holiday, an interval between childhood and manhood, before they reverted for ever to the social or hereditary type to which at heart they belonged. Bertrand Russell once defined a gentleman as someone whose great grandparents had £1000 a year. In this sense, all my friends at Oxford were gentlemen, and they bore the marks of it inescapably, just as I did not.

"You never know what anyone's really like until you've met his brother," someone once said to me; he meant that, in most cases, differences of personality are superficial compared with the underlying similarities which are the product of social and family environment. And in this sense my friends and acquaintances at Oxford could truly be said to have belonged to one large family, which, however many and varied its branches, impressed upon all its members certain distinguishing marks which they all shared, just as every Spanish Hapsburg shared an hereditary tendency to haemophilia. For the same reason, there operated in them a certain principle of exclusiveness towards all who, whether by descent or adoption, did not share the same tribal affinities. The little world of Oxford, though within its own limits it offered the most generous opportunities for the development of the individual, nevertheless excluded far more than it embraced.

As time went by, I began to feel a kind of dissatisfaction because, just as Oxford had once seemed to offer a wider world than Wales, so it began to seem that beyond its walls there lay even larger possibilities, which might indeed be a jungle as compared with its cultivated garden, but where nothing survived except at the cost of a struggle against which Oxford offered all too adequate a protection. My dissatisfaction was muted because of the generosity with which Oxford opened its arms to me. It was not the individual which she excluded but only the social and intellectual forms which were not compatible with her own assumptions. From one point of view it was a closed city; but from another it was an open-ended one, in the sense that anyone might enter it who had the means and the wish to, and Oxford made his entry easy, with all the grace of a bountiful mother who, already endowed with plenty of children of her own, is always happy and willing to adopt more. The Oxford of my day was certainly the creation, in many ways a beautiful one, of a highly developed class system; but it was also a gate which was open to anyone who had the necessary entrance ticket.

It was also the corridor by which the ticket holders might pass, on favourable terms, into the adult world for which Oxford was a preparation. They would become civil servants, judges, politicians, bankers, soldiers, dons, doctors, scientists, schoolmasters; they were officer cadets in the great army of legislators, administrators and executives required to rule Britain and its empire, which still covered a third of the world's surface. There was even room in the system for writers and artists, and some of my friends, and those I liked the best, had already decided that this was to be theirs; they did so with an assurance which amazed me that for them also society would provide. Nor did those who, out of natural idealism, had formed the hope, and the intention, of changing, even overturning, society, feel excluded from its benefits; somehow they assumed that society itself would provide them with the means of achieving its own reform, and that the labyrinth of the British constitution had its own signposts which would lead them to the minotaur they wished to slay.

There was another confidence which my contemporaries shared. It was the confidence that the adult world which they were soon to enter would essentially reproduce the pattern of relationships which they had learned at Oxford, and that among them the personal connections they had formed at Oxford would continue to play an important part. Society would continue to bring them together, their paths in life would continue to cross, and this in itself would be part of the machinery through which society would exercise its functions. It was a justified assumption because Oxford foreshadowed the adult world as an embryo foreshadows the grown man; all the elements were there which would later be operative in the society which my contemporaries would administer together. Of course, not all expectations would be fulfilled. Some would rise higher than others, and it was a popular after-dinner pastime to compose lists of those most likely to succeed; the laws of probability made it statistically certain that many of those at Oxford then were bound to succeed greatly and it was only a question of picking out whom the wheel of fortune would carry highest. Others would falter by the wayside, some would sink into decent obscurity. But somehow it was always assumed that all would continue to exist on the same terms of easy familiarity as they had learned at Oxford, that the channels of communication established there would always remain open, that friendships once founded would never quite fail, and that the fine web of relationships of which Oxford was the centre would always permit even them some degree of influence on the society of which they were the privileged class.

I do not know whether it was simply my origins and upbringing, or something else in me, which prevented me from making the same confident assumption about my own future. Perhaps it was the latter, because in the case of my brother I could see no reason why, having proceeded from Aberystwyth to Cambridge, he should not continue his progress to an assured place in the English Establishment. There was a sense in which I loved Oxford; but it was more like a passing infatuation than a lifetime's affection. With the best will in the world, I could not see myself at home in the world to which Oxford was the natural entry; the trouble was that I could not see myself at home in any other either. On the whole, it seemed to me that chance, luck, Providence or misfortune had led me to Oxford, without much collaboration from me, and that I should do better to trust whatever mysterious power had been at work than to interfere with its operations by any initiative of my own.

Such a view was all the more persuasive because the will, it seemed, was a faculty in which I was almost totally deficient. It showed itself, at most, only in a stubborn determination to have my own way in anything that concerned my own pleasure, but it was apparently incapable of implementing any coherent or consistent plan for the future. It may have been some vestigial remains of my father's Augustinian theology which so convinced me that no deliberate purpose of mine would have any effect on what happened to me; I looked on myself as the child of some inscrutable power compounded of grace and chance, a ball on some cosmic roulette wheel on which the same number never turned up twice. Sometimes I had the curious sensation that the most I could do was to bet on where it would fall next, without any power of affecting the result. Nor was I particularly anxious to, though some rudimentary sense of self-preservation warned me that I should be making some kind of preparation for the future. My own expectations varied with whether at any particular moment euphoria or depression was in the ascendant. In moments of elation, which were many, I felt I could not do better than to trust in the luck which had carried me to Oxford; in moods of gloom, which were no less frequent, I felt that whatever turn the wheel of fortune should take next, it could only be for the worse; in either case, I felt, there was nothing I could do about it.

Thus I felt that my existence at Oxford was a strictly provisional and transitional one, in the sense especially that neither Oxford nor the society which had produced it could provide any settled habitation for me. This was an all-pervading sense, that applied to every aspect of life at Oxford; but it was accentuated by one particular aspect which more than anything else distinguished it from anything with which I had hitherto been familiar.

There were very many things which at that time made Oxford a very different place from the world outside its walls; ease, comfort, freedom from material pressures, intellectual opportunities, friendship, access to almost any of the pleasures which most satisfied one's tastes. These were genuine privileges, even luxuries, and one was lucky to enjoy them; one would have been ungrateful indeed if one did not. But it had one distinctive feature which, for me at least, almost cancelled all its other advantages. For Oxford was at that time, in a way it has long ceased to be, an almost exclusively male society, from which the *ewig Weibliche* was totally absent, both in the spirit and the flesh, and this made life there even more abnormal, one might even say unnatural, than it would otherwise have been. Women of course did physically exist there, both in the town and, on its dim outskirts, in the women's colleges, but in the life of the university they exerted little or no influence; so far as most undergraduates were concerned they might just as well not have existed.

This was not so much through force of circumstances, but as a matter of choice. Women undergraduates were indeed few in number at that time, but it was not so much their number, or lack of them, which counted. It was that they were second-class citizens in the hierarchy of the university, whose activities, whether serious or frivolous, were organized entirely for the satisfaction of masculine tastes; except, that is to say, of that one taste which in most men, and particularly young men, is one of the most dominant and powerful.

In Oxford, on the other hand, it seemed to be almost entirely in abeyance, as if, for most undergraduates, normal biological laws had been for the time being suspended. In this sense, Oxford was for them merely a continuation of the conditions under which they had lived at their public schools, where, willy nilly, their emotional and sexual instincts could find no personal objects of satisfaction except in each other. For most of them, by the time they came to Oxford, this had come to seem the natural condition of human life and it was natural that at the university they should, like well-conditioned animals, persevere in the habits and the attitudes to which they had been trained at school. Nor, on the whole, was there anyone to teach them otherwise. Universities are not designed to be schools of sexual therapy; and in any case dons, for the most part, were then precisely those who as adults remained happy with the same range of emotional satisfactions that they had known as schoolboys and undergraduates.

It might be said that most undergraduates, and their elders, at Oxford in those days lived in a state of sexual infantilism. It pervaded the entire life of the university, giving it a peculiar colour and flavour of its own, which accentuated even further the differences between life within and without its walls; it was as if some thousands of young men lived under conditions which, in one important respect at least, approximated to those of the nursery. What was more remarkable was that to most of them this was quite imperceptible, as if, in such matters, they were colour blind or their taste buds had not developed. To them, the notion that men should live without women was perfectly natural; to some, even, it was the only acceptable way of life. It was the idea that women are an essential and indispensable part of a man's existence which struck them as abnormal and bizarre; indeed, as an undergraduate, I was sometimes rebuked for deliberate eccentricity or gross exaggeration when I ventured to assert such a proposition, which to me was self-evident.

Yet men, especially young men, do not deprive themselves of the company of women without undergoing a modification of their whole nature, often in ways so subtle and pervasive that they themselves are hardly aware of it; in particular, their capacity for feeling and emotion is turned upon each other and not, as they would be otherwise in the great majority of cases, towards members of the opposite sex. I do not mean by this that men without women necessarily become homosexual in the direct and simple sense of that word, nor that most undergraduates in my time were homosexual in that sense, though a large number certainly were and almost aggressively so; perhaps indeed it was they who had the best of it. I mean rather that under such conditions what men love and admire most is formed in the male image and not its opposite, that their ideas, their affections, even their intimations of good and evil are exclusively expressed in the masculine gender, and that it is in the man, that is to say themselves, that they find their deepest aspirations realized. For them, the Fall was an event that only happened to Eve; only she was expelled, and Adam was left to enjoy the garden alone with the serpent.

Some such version of the Biblical legend might have served very well as a description of Oxford in my time. Oxford, with its towers and spires, its cupolas and pinnacles, its river-bounded meadows and elm-tree walks, its ancient stones that crumbled and flaked beneath one's fingers, might very well have served in those days as an image of Paradise, but it was a paradise which was men's exclusive preserve. It followed that their pleasures and passions were directed towards each other, and this gave what might well have seemed to others an exaggerated intensity to the experiences which they shared together. Perhaps this helps to explain the kind of golden haze which envelops, or once enveloped, many people's reminiscences of Oxford, as a kind of land of lost content in which, given the peculiar nature of their education, they did what came most naturally to them. It was what came after that seemed a fall from grace.

In some cases, of course, this attitude took an overtly sexual form, and they were the more conspicuous because they included some of the most gifted of my contemporaries, both among undergraduates and dons. For many, homosexuality was simply a fashion; to the committed homosexual it was a creed and a cult, with its own rituals which were hidden from the profane. It was also a standard which could be brandished bravely in the great war between the Hearties and the Aesthetes, it was the flag of culture as opposed to philistinism, and it was also a symbol of that intense cultivation of personal relations in which Oxford placed so much faith. Moreover, it was a flag of rebellion; to be homosexual was at once the easiest and most flagrant way of affronting the moral values of Bird's Custard Island and for many it served the same purpose as drug addiction today.

But such active standard-bearers of the cause of homo-sexuality, precursors of the hippies and dropouts of today, were, like them, very much in a minority. What was characteristic of the Oxford scene was the prevalence, even in those who were least aware of it, of an attitude of mind and heart which took it for granted that the deepest emotional satisfactions were only to be found in a mas-culine society, and that any others could never be anything better than second-rate; it was an attitude which not only conditioned their behaviour at Oxford, their relations with each other, their ideas of what is best and worst in the world, but continued to do so long after they had gone down and had become the most respectable of citizens and fathers of families. Whether such an attitude is properly to be called homosexual I do not know; but it was an attitude which profoundly affected an entire generation of middle-class Englishmen of the governing class, and even today has not entirely vanished.

It was all the more striking to me because, as I thought, I could trace a clear relationship between this underlying prejudice in favour of the male, which was characteristic of the most normal undergraduate, and the more overt and ostentatious manifestations of homosexuality. These, in the more extreme cases, sometimes took the form of affectations in dress which clearly proclaimed their wearer's sexual loyalties, or in a particular manner of gesture, gait and physical comportment whose significance was no less unmistakeable. Sometimes they combined to create creatures who paraded through the streets of Oxford like brightly plumaged birds of paradise, attract-ing the attention of all by their flamboyant costume, their high-pitched cries, their quick, elusive movements. But these after all were only the outward and visible signs of an inward emotional commitment which was shared by Oxford society as a whole, even though the great majority of undergraduates would never have dreamed of indulging in such extravagances. It was a commitment which in Oxford's sister university of Cambridge had, under the influence of a long and distinguished line of teachers and moralists achieved the status of a philosophy, explicitly in the writings of G. E. Moore and implicitly in the novels of E. M. Forster, and more especially in Forster's famous pronouncement: "Only connect". It could be said that those two words, so seductive in their simplicity, so misleading in their ambiguity, had more influence in shaping the emotional attitudes of the English governing class between the two world wars than any other single phrase in the English language.

Oxford at the end of the twenties had no such great names to give moral authority to its predilection for the male over the female principle, or its belief that intense personal relations between persons of the same sex embody one of the highest moral values. Compared with Cambridge, Oxford was intellectually indolent in its approach to such matters; practice, not philosophy, was what it was interested in. But the two universities were bound together by an elaborate network of relationships, historical, institutional and personal; both drew their undergraduates from the same social class; and both sent them out to rule England and its empire imprinted with the belief that life would never have anything better to offer than the kind of relationships they had enjoyed with each other at the university.

I do not know whether such an education so narrowly based upon class and the domination of the male worked for their own good or, later, for the good of the country and the empire which to all intents and purposes they governed and administered up to the end of the Second World War. The history of England between the wars suggests that on the whole it did not. But I certainly derived far too much pleasure from the company of my friends at Oxford to wish that they should have been otherwise than what they were, or that education had made them different. But they came at the end of a long historical and intellectual tradition, itself the product of very exceptional social conditions, which at that moment was very rapidly running into the sands. It was not, I think, on the whole a good thing that young men designed and destined to form the executive and governing class of a great country should have received their higher education at institutions which were a combination of a monastery and a nursery. In this particular respect Oxford, and Cambridge also, at the end of the 1920s had advanced very little beyond the Middle Ages. Its products were still, as then, in essence clerks whose future lay in supplying church and state with the staff required to operate their administrative machines; and in effect they still, as then, subscribed to the rule of celibacy which applied to the medieval clerk. Only that rule no longer derived its authority from the love of God, but, rather, from the kind of love which David had for Jonathan, a love surpassing the love of women; and to that kind of affection, in all its many variations, they attached an importance and value which were as near absolute as anything could be.

As for me, my instincts rebelled against such a system of values, even though I might accidentally profit by it, and I felt that in such a society there was not likely to be much of a place for me. It was not that I regarded it with horror or aversion. It was simply that I believed it rested

on false intellectual and emotional foundations, and
somehow this seemed to involve yet another division
between my friends and myself. Public schools were bad
enough; it was even worse if they were to provide the
standards for adult life. I felt reinforced in my instinctive
feeling that Oxford was not for me nor I for Oxford.

III

I am aware that what I have written applies almost
entirely to an Oxford which no longer exists, and that the
Oxford of today bears little or no resemblance to Oxford
as it was then, any more than I do to the young man I
was as an undergraduate; both might be said to have died
together. So far as Oxford is concerned, much of the
change was due to the great expansion of the university
which took place after the Second World War, and not
less to social and industrial changes which have totally
destroyed that sense of intimacy and privacy which was
once an essential part of Oxford's charm, just as they have
totally transformed the character of its academic population. But the change had begun even before I myself
ceased to be an undergraduate, and the Oxford of the
1930s was already not the place that I had known when
I first went there in 1928.

The distinguishing mark of Oxford when I first knew
it was a kind of enlightened pursuit of pleasure. This
gave Oxford a certain air of frivolity and gaiety which
was in itself highly agreeable; but it was also compatible,
in those for whom ideas were the greatest of all diversions,
with a genuine devotion to learning for its own sake.
Indeed, I am not sure that true learning, so opposed to
what is today called research, can flourish in any other
kind of air. This particular combination of frivolity with
the pursuit of knowledge was something in which young

men, according to their capacity, were very privileged to share, because it was unlikely that they would ever come across it again anywhere else; it had something of that *douceur de vie* which Talleyrand ascribed to the *ancien régime* before the French Revolution. It was the product of the late last flowering of an empire which was already in decay, but was still strong enough and wealthy enough to support a class which was largely immune to the pressure of material care and could afford to devote itself to pursuits which from one point of view were an extreme form of conspicuous waste but from another were essential to a humane and liberal education. Its existence was made possible by the vast wealth accumulated by Britain in over a century of triumphant material progress; the hoard had been appreciably diminished by the First World War, but it was still very large and still sufficient to maintain Oxford as a kind of seminary/nursery/playground for its privileged youth. Not many of them, at that time, made the direct connection between their privileges and what went on beyond the walls of Oxford; most of them took it for granted that this was as things were and as they would continue to be and, this being so, why should they not continue with the cultivation of their own personal tastes which, consciously in some cases, unconsciously in others, was their main preoccupation at Oxford?

But already, while I was an undergraduate, the first warning shadows, like the first touches of evening, fell across the scene. The first, perhaps, in the spring of 1929, was the collapse of the considerable financial empire created by the great embezzler Clarence Hatry. This, though it shook the City of London and some have attributed to it a considerable influence on the great slump that was to follow, made no great impression on Oxford; but it had considerable repercussions among the class which provided Oxford with its recruits, and at least two of my acquaintances disappeared before their time as a result. Of far greater significance, in the Michaelmas term of 1929, at the beginning of my second year at Oxford, and shortly before my twentieth birthday, was the great stock exchange collapse on Wall Street, which, with its consequences, was to affect the lives of an entire generation, in ways which would have been unthinkable only a year before. At first it went unnoticed, even by those who, like myself, were supposed to be interested in economics; my economics tutor, in reply to my enquiries, assured me that it was a purely superficial stock exchange phenomenon, that would have no effect except the healthy one of shaking out the lunatic fringe of the great Wall Street boom. But in fact it was the beginning of the great economic depression of the 30s, which convulsed the capitalist world and led to the triumph of Hitler in Germany and finally to the Second World War.

In such a world there was no room for Oxford as I had first known it. Increasingly, the eyes and minds of undergraduates were directed to events that were taking place beyond her walls, and particularly in Germany, where the Weimar Republic, the home of so many *avant garde* experiments in the arts and in morals, was entering its death throes. As the depression deepened, and capitalism seemed helpless either to remedy it or to alleviate the sufferings it inflicted, it transformed Adolf Hitler from an *opera bouffe* Bavarian politician into a world figure of nightmare proportions, and his triumph in Germany was the prelude to a series of political disasters that followed one another with the inevitability of a Greek tragedy. This tragedy was enacted against a background which was occupied by a vast, grey army of workless men, whose existence seemed both to threaten the capitalist system and to make a mockery of it as a method of satisfying human needs. Some of their bitterness and frustration spilled over even into Oxford, when the long shabby columns of the Hunger Marchers shuffled into the city, to be fed in soup kitchens and put to rest in whatever shelter could be found for them. For many undergraduates, it was the first time that they had ever seen a hungry man with their own eyes.

It is to the credit of undergraduates of a younger generation than mine that, as economic and political conditions deteriorated, they became increasingly concerned with the world outside Oxford and with efforts to avert the catastrophies which lay ahead. In this they followed a humane and generous instinct. It was not from any sense of self-preservation that they flung themselves into political agitation and debate, because they did not really feel that they were themselves directly threatened; it was rather out of sympathy with the victims of the economic depression and the rise of fascism, which made it impossible for the young and generous in spirit to ignore the ugly realities of the world outside. But such feelings put an end, perhaps rightly, to the kind of society which had existed in Oxford during the 1920s. Love of the arts, sexual experiment, personal relationships, delight in the many-coloured surface of life, seemed a poor and inhuman response to the sufferings of millions of men and women. Pleasure gave way to politics; aesthetes and homosexuals suddenly turned revolutionaries, political agitation took the place of dinner parties and conversation gave way to polemics. Voices grew shrill, and the masses took the place of the individual as the object of reverence and respect; undergraduates awoke to the fact that even in Britain there were three million men and their families who were near the starvation line and that there actually existed in the world, especially in Germany, bad men possessed by an evil will which could not be constrained except by force. Moral and political indignation persuaded them that the time had come to change the world instead of enjoying it. In the eyes of many undergraduates, Oxford, so encumbered with the remains of a past which had given birth to the horrors of the present, had suddenly ceased to be a pleasure garden and become an Ivory Tower, whose only function was to provide an escape from the catastrophies of the "real" world.

In Cambridge, this revulsion against the comforts, amenities, and intellectual delights of the academic *hortus conclusus* was even more violent than at Oxford, just as its analysis of its system of values had been more refined. There, some of the brightest and best of their generation, like Guy Burgess or Kim Philby, totally committed themselves to forms of political action which in fact were even worse than the evils they were intended to avert, with results which, many years later, were to astonish the world. Oxford, on the whole, did not go as far as this; even in her conversion to politics there remained, for most of the converts, a certain residue of dilettantism, of worldly wisdom, which forbade total sacrifice or martyrdom. But even at Oxford political commitment, however muddleheaded or even farcical it sometimes was, went far enough to destroy the university as I first knew it. The left wing political generation of the 1930s may not have had much success in their efforts to change the world; but they certainly transformed Oxford out of all recognition.

IV

When at length the time came for me to go down from Oxford, it found me in a mood compounded of gloom and relief; gloom, because I had no idea of what was going to happen to me, and felt a certain apprehension that it might not be very pleasant, certainly nothing like so pleasant as the three years I had just passed; relief, because I had begun to feel that the time for those particular pleasures was over, and that beyond Oxford events were taking place which somehow made them look trivial and unimportant.

On the last day of term, when the college was already deserted, I walked with a friend round New College gardens. His future was decided, and after the vacation he was proceeding to Paris to study for the entrance examination for the diplomatic service. The evening was grey and chilly, with that air of damp and melancholy which seems to settle in Oxford at almost any season of the year. A cold wind ruffled the branches of the trees; it seemed as if autumn had already come. My final examinations were over and I had the sense of having performed very indifferently; twinges of conscience for so many wasted hours, guilt at having disappointed my parents' expectations, afflicted me intermittently like an infected tooth. My own prospects seemed unbelievably bleak and depressing, and those last hours in the garden had a dull note of finality because, however the future might turn out, I was quite sure that it was not likely to bring me back to Oxford. I felt as if I were looking at it all for the last time: the green lawns, the city walls that enclosed the garden, the tree-grown mound on which King Charles had mounted his cannon to bombard Cromwell's army, the little Norman tower of St Peter's-in-the-East where Walter Pater lay buried; I was quite sure that I should not see any of it again.

Of course, I was quite wrong, as my expectations of the future have always proved to be; manic-depressive types suffer such regular alternations of mood that the fears or hopes they form in one stage of the cycle are never, for good or bad, realized in the next one. When the results of my final examinations appeared, I was surprised and pleased to find that I had after all been given a First, though candid friends also informed me that it had been a very close thing. My philosophy tutor ended his letter of congratulation enigmatically with the words: "So I hope you have learned a lesson; and the *Right Lesson!*" I was not at all sure what the Right Lesson might be, but the letter effectively disposed of any satisfaction I might have felt at the result. It was quite clear that it was not merit, it was luck, that had been at work.

That summer my mother died, as if, having sent me to Oxford and received the news of my success, there was nothing more for her to do. It was the worst single thing that has ever happened to me, and it left me dazed and bewildered, as if it were totally beyond my apprehension. Its effect was all the worse because at night, in the neighbouring bedroom, I could hear my father crying out her name in his sleep.

Unless one is a singularly pure character, grief, especially when compounded with guilt, confuses all one's reactions; one does not know how to respond to a situation for which one had deliberately contrived not to prepare oneself. My mother's death, that summer, deprived me of any power to make a rational decision about the future. Without my mother, indeed, the future seemed to be a concept that had no meaning. I simply took what came along, which happened to be an offer of a senior scholarship at New College, which would make it possible for me to return to Oxford for another year to read history. I accepted it rather in the spirit of a doomed man who sees no alternative to execution, for my other scholarships had now come to an end, and I did not really see how I was to survive a year at Oxford on an income of £120 a year. But there seemed nothing else to do, so that having in June said farewell to Oxford for ever, I found myself back there once again some three months later, looking for rooms in which to spend the coming academic year.

Once again chance took a hand. My history tutor during my last year was a Fellow of All Souls; meeting me in the street as I pursued my searches, he took me to lunch at the college and suggested I should sit for its fellowship examination, which was to take place shortly. There did not seem much point in doing so, but he was encouraging and persuasive; in any case, as he said, I had nothing to lose, and even to fail the examination is a kind of distinction of its own. So I followed his suggestion, went through the somewhat bewildering series of trials which All Souls imposes on candidates for its prize fellowships, and on All Souls' Day, November 2, while I was lunching with some friends in my rooms, I was astounded to be waited upon by a servant from All Souls and informed that I had been elected to a fellowship and would be expected, in my new-found capacity, to dine in the college that night. So it seemed as if Oxford had not yet done with me. There were some children playing in the street outside my windows. I collected all the money I had in my rooms or could borrow from my guests and in an expansive gesture of gratitude scattered it from the window and watched the children as they tried to catch the coins as they fell or chased them along the pavement and the gutters.

v

In those days a prize fellowship at All Souls was regarded as one of the greatest gifts Oxford had to bestow, and a sure guarantee of success in whatever career one chose to adopt. When I was elected, the college included among its forty members one archbishop, one bishop, an ex-Viceroy of India, several cabinet ministers, the two brightest luminaries of the English bar, and the editor of *The Times* (an office which had become almost hereditary in the college). I was not the first product of the state system of education to be elected to the college, but I was certainly the first Welsh one, and in Wales itself my election was regarded as a matter for national self-congratulation. It was a matter of grief to me that my mother was not alive to know of it; she would have regarded it as the culmination of all the ambitions she had cherished for me, but it was some compensation that it was a considerable source of pride to my father.

On the other hand, perhaps perversely, to me my election was, and remained, a source of guilt; partly because I thought I detected in it once again the hand of chance or luck, and also because I felt it identified me with a way of life which was opposed to everything which I desired. For I too had succumbed to the wave of radical political feeling which was beginning to sweep through the universities. It confirmed me in the socialist ideas which I had cherished since my schooldays, and now, as the depression deepened, and its consequences became increasingly evident, it began to seem as if any day the hour of revolution might be at hand. The year was 1931, which Arnold Toynbee called the *Annus Terribilis*, when government after government was falling under the impact of the depression; the walls of the capitalist Jericho seemed to be crumbling before one's very eyes.

It seemed absurd, at such a moment, to find oneself safely and comfortably installed at the very heart of the Establishment, all the more so because this meant, in my case, occupying in his absence the rooms of Sir John Simon, then Secretary of State for Foreign Affairs. I used to go through his wardrobe and finger, and sometimes even wear in cold weather, the excellent thick striped flannel shirts in which it abounded. My condition was even worse, it seemed to me, because the college welcomed one, as a junior fellow on such easy and generous terms that they really left one nothing to rebel against; there was only the conviction that the college, with its narrow Hawksmoor towers, its Wren sundial, its beautiful view of the dome of the Radcliffe Camera poised like a marvellous bubble outside its gates, represented the kingdom of this world which was about to be punished for its sins, and which, in any case, it was the duty of any good Calvinist or socialist to reject.

The emoluments of a prize fellow were then £300 a year, with free rooms and a free dinner, and if one chose to drink, as I did, one did so at ludicrously cheap rates which were heavily subsidized by the college. To me this was a fortune, and despite my socialism, it only slightly marred my enjoyment of it that an unemployed family in South Wales lived on 30/– a week. But it was not only the material comforts which were felt as a source of potential corruption. The college was a very small community, of whose members only a very few were at any moment in residence. There were no undergraduates to disturb the *luxe, calme, et volupté* of the fellows; one lived as if in some retired country house, its peace only broken by the dim hum of traffic in the High, and sometimes, at night, walking its corridors and staircase while the college slept and outside the moonlight turned to silver the leaden dome of the Radcliffe, one could imagine that one was its sole proprietor and only the dead surrounded one.

It was all the more pleasant because the house was

supplied with every facility for the pursuit of learning, even if no one very much bothered whether one made use of them; and because one lived on the easiest and most comfortable terms with its other residents. All of them were older than myself, most of them very much older, and some were men of great distinction and achievement; but all had the gift of treating one as if one were their equal, and a bishop or a cabinet minister listened to one with the same patience and attention as if one were a bishop or cabinet minister oneself. All Souls indeed repeated in an even more concentrated form the same lesson I had learned at New College; that once accepted by the ruling class there is none of their privileges which they will not willingly and gladly share with you. The only difficulty was that I could not accept myself in such company.

Otherwise, life was very agreeable and to me all the more so because, for two years at least, a prize fellowship seemed to entail practically no duties whatsoever. For those two years, out of the seven for which one was initially elected, it was assumed that one was still continuing a course of initiation into an adult life which had not yet really begun. After all, once a fellow one's future was in some sense assured, there was no need to hurry, there was time to make mistakes and to pursue false scents; the serious business of life could be postponed for a few years longer. In the meantime, as the youngest and most junior fellow, it was my duty to prepare the salad before dinner, and in common room after dinner, as Mister Screw, to decant the port.

Some of this was explained to me when, the morning after my election, and having celebrated it by drinking rather too much the night before, I waited upon the Warden of All Souls in his study. He might have been taken as a model for a scholar and a gentleman of the old school, to whom all mundane cares were both alien and distasteful, but he was in fact an eminently practical, if slightly idle, man of affairs. A moderate classical scholar, for a time a moderately successful barrister, a moderately good administrator whose motto was above all *pas trop de zèle*, he was admirably suited to his position and it to him, all the more so because the long Oxford vacations allowed him to spend a large part of his time on his estates in Shropshire; he had the fresh pink cheeks of a country squire who spends many hours in the open air without exposing himself to its harsher elements. I was not sure whether I could not also detect a hint of something slightly sly, almost shifty, in his faded blue eyes.

To me that morning he was kindness itself. He enquired politely about my schooling and my career as an undergraduate, and when I had told him everything I thought it proper for him to know, he surprised me by saying: "You must have worked very hard."

My tutor's complaint, it had seemed to me, was precisely that I had not worked very hard, and I was inclined to agree with him; all the same, I was touched by the Warden's perception that perhaps, after all, there had been a good deal of effort involved.

"It's not easy to take the fellowship examination straight after your schools," he went on. "What are you thinking of doing now?"

I said that I had very little idea. I had intended to take the history school in my additional year at Oxford, but now that seemed rather pointless.

"I should think a rest would be good for you," he said kindly.

It had not occurred to me that this was what I needed, but somehow it was pleasant to be told that it was.

"Go abroad perhaps. Look at some pictures. Go to the

opera." The last words were spoken almost wistfully, as if they represented some almost unattainable peak of happiness. I suddenly began to feel that the Warden was a man after my own heart. If there was anything I wanted it was to be away from Oxford and from academic life, to be "abroad", which seemed to have not so much a geographical as a spiritual connotation. I said that I wanted to go to Vienna and to Berlin, to improve my German and also of course to enjoy those delights which the Warden held out to me as if they were his to dispose of; but also, though I did not mention this, because I thought that in Germany and Austria revolutionary events were at hand.

"A very good idea," the Warden said heartily. "Only of course you'll have to pernoctate." This meant that the statutes of the college required that a prize fellow had to spend a given number of nights in college during an academic year. It was not a heavy burden; if I spent three months in Oxford I could go away for at least a year.

We drank a glass of sherry before we left. It was a cold November day and my head was aching, yet the sun seemed to be shining brightly, as if some totally new prospect of the future had suddenly been revealed to me. And somehow, both on that day and in later years, it seemed to me that Oxford would never again mean to me what it had meant before.

Three

In fact, I did not go abroad until later than I expected. Life was very pleasant at All Souls, and I thought I had better prepare myself for the task I projected for myself in Germany, which was to write a biography of the great politician and demagogue, friend of Marx and Engels, and founder of the German Social Democratic party, Ferdinand Lassalle. I regarded the prospect with some apprehension; I felt that the walls of the academic prison house were beginning to close around me and yet struggled only feebly to escape them. All that could come later, I thought.

It was at the beginning of the summer term of 1932 that I first met a visiting Cambridge undergraduate called Guy Burgess. He was staying for the weekend with Maurice Bowra, who was then Dean of Wadham and, during my undergraduate life, had probably influenced me more than anyone else at Oxford. I had heard of Guy before, because he had the reputation of being the most brilliant undergraduate of his day at Cambridge, and I looked forward to his visit with some interest.

We met at a dinner party given by Felix Frankfurter who was then a visiting professor at Oxford, and Guy and I immediately made great friends. Indeed, he did not belie his reputation. He was then a scholar of Trinity, and it was thought that he had a brilliant academic future in front of him. That evening he talked a good deal about painting and to me it seemed that what he said was both original and sensitive, and, for one so young, to show an unusually wide knowledge of the object. His conversation had the more charm because he was very good looking in a boyish, athletic, very English way; it seemed incongruous that almost everything he said made it quite clear that he was a homosexual and a communist.

After dinner, though it was late, we walked back to All Souls together, and I took him into the deserted smoking room, where we drank whisky together for a long time. At first he made tentative amorous advances, but quickly and cheerfully desisted when he discovered that I was as heterosexual as he was the opposite; he would have done the same to any young man, because sex to him was both a compulsion and a game which it was almost a duty to practise. He went on to talk about painting, and its relation to the Marxist interpretation of history, and about the busmen's strike which he was helping to organize in Cambridge; it seemed to me that there was something deeply original, something which was, as it were, his very own, in everything he had to say. It was not that the matters he talked about were unusual; by 1932 they had become topics of almost incessant discussion by the intellectual-homosexual-aesthetic-communist young man who was rapidly establishing himself as the classical, and fashionable, type of progressive undergraduate.

To such a young man, Marxism and communism were something to be argued about, debated, elucidated, defended; it was something which lay outside the bounds of his experience, and remained an opinion or a faith to be held with a greater or less degree of conviction. For Guy it was simply a way of looking at the world which seemed as natural to him as the way he breathed. It was a kind of category of thought, like the Kantian categories of time and space, which was fundamental to the way in which he perceived and apprehended the world. This was something which I never met among Guy's, or my, English,

contemporaries who, during the 1930s, adopted communism as an intellectual creed; somehow there always
remained in them an assimilated residuum of their liberal
upbringing which was in conflict with the faith they
professed. In Guy such a conflict seemed to have been
entirely resolved; in this respect at least he never changed
through all the years I knew him, so that, whatever the
vagaries of his conduct or his professions, I somehow
took it for granted that fundamentally he always remained
a communist, even if, for reasons of his own, he chose to
deny it. Marxism had entered so deeply into him that he
simply could not think in any other way. This is a
characteristic which I came later to recognize in professional communists whom I met in Germany and Austria,
but never, so far as I am aware, in any English ones.

During his weekend visit Guy and I liked each other
well enough to make tentative plans to visit the Soviet
Union during the summer vacation. For some reason
these came to nothing as far as I was concerned, and Guy
took as his companion a young undergraduate from
Balliol, who was also both communist and homosexual.
He gave me a vivid account of Guy lying dead drunk in
the Park of Rest and Culture in Moscow; otherwise I
could not discover much of what went on. Guy described
to me a long discussion he had had with Nikolai Bukharin,
ex-secretary of the Comintern, ex-editor of *Pravda* and
later to be executed by Stalin, and treated me to a long
and brilliant disquisition on the pictures in the Hermitage.
Otherwise I never knew him to talk about his experiences
in the Soviet Union, and I do not think they ever
affected his beliefs one way or another. It was as if his
communism formed a closed intellectual system which
had nothing to do with what actually went on in the
socialist fatherland. If one had pointed out to him that at

the moment of his visit the Soviet Union was recovering from a profound economic crisis and was now entering a period of violent political reaction, he would have regarded it as being, even if true, irrelevant.

Side by side with his political activities, Guy conducted a very active, very promiscuous and somewhat squalid sexual life. He was gross and even brutal in his treatment of his lovers, but his sexual behaviour also had a generous aspect. He was very attractive to his own sex and had none of the kind of inhibitions which were then common to young men of his age, class and education. He regarded sex as a useful machine for the manufacture of pleasure, and perhaps for this reason was very successful in satisfying his appetites. In this he was unlike his friends at Cambridge, who were nearly all homosexual but a good deal more timid than Guy, a good deal more frustrated, and a good deal less successful in their sexual adventures, which on the whole were coloured by sentimental and emotional overtones which to Guy were simply absurd. At one time or another he went to bed with most of these friends, as he did with anyone who was willing and was not positively repulsive, and in doing so he released them from many of their frustrations and inhibitions. He was a kind of public schoolboy's guide to the mysteries of sex, and he fulfilled his function almost with a sense of public service. Such affairs did not last for long; but Guy had the faculty of retaining the affection of those he went to bed with, and also, in some curious way, of maintaining a kind of permanent domination over them. This was strengthened because, long after the affair was over, he continued to assist his friends in their sexual lives, which were often troubled and unsatisfactory, to listen to their emotional difficulties and when necessary find suitable partners for them. To such people he was a combination of father confessor and pimp, and the number of people who were under an obligation to him for the kind of services which the confessor and pimp can supply must have been very large indeed.

I learned all this from Guy himself, who spoke of such activities with a kind of amused candour, from which any sense of shame was entirely lacking; no doubt he thought that such frankness was more likely to provoke my interest than my disapproval. Indeed, he seemed to take a delight in offering one, as if for inspection, the psychological puzzles in which his character abounded. One could not help wondering whether the services he performed for his friends were genuinely given, as they themselves believed, out of altruism, or whether they were the result of some conscious or unconscious wish to dominate. The second alternative seemed the more likely; he saw himself sometimes as a kind of Figaro figure, ever resourceful in the service of others in order to manipulate them to his own ends.

Such a possibility only occurred to me many years after I first met him, when the contradictions in his character and behaviour seemed to have become so acute as to be insoluble. While I was still an undergraduate I had driven over to Cambridge with a young don, for whom the main object of the visit had been to visit Guy, with whom he was at the time in love. When, long after, I reminded Guy of the incident he laughed and said he remembered it very well, and then added: "And indeed I still have his letters." I thought that perhaps he was boasting; but after a search through the incredible disorder of his rooms he produced a neat little bundle of letters labelled with the name of the enamoured don.

I had known already that Guy never destroyed a letter but had simply put this down as yet another among the many oddities in his character. But that he deliberately preserved them and that somewhere there might exist an enormous accumulation of letters, neatly filed and docketed, from his former lovers had never occurred to me. Certainly it was not affection which had prompted the preservation of this particular bundle of letters; but what other motive could there be? I must confess that for a moment I contemplated with a kind of horrified fascination the power which such a collection might confer upon its possessor and of the jeopardy in which they might conceivably place those who had written them. But then, as so often with Guy, I put the idea aside as far-fetched and exaggerated; the trouble was, I thought, that he stimulated my imagination too much. It was only a kind of magpie instinct which prevented him from destroying even the most trivial piece of correspondence.

II

After that summer, in which I saw Guy frequently, I went abroad, and on my return went to work in Manchester as a leader writer on the *Manchester Guardian*. For the next two years I saw little or nothing of Guy, but I heard of him from friends we had in common and it seemed that the bright confident morning of his undergraduate days had begun to fade. In particular, he had failed to fulfil the promise of a brilliant academic career, or indeed of any particular kind of career at all. In his third year at Cambridge he had suffered a severe nervous breakdown and had taken an *aegrotat* degree; nevertheless, he returned to Cambridge with the intention of submitting a thesis for a fellowship at Trinity. At this point he was still an open and active member of the communist party; shortly afterwards, however, in circumstances of great publicity, even scandal, so far as the confined world of Cambridge was concerned, he quarrelled ostentatiously with his communist friends and even his more liberal-minded ones, and left Cambridge for London.

The effects of Guy's rupture with the communist party reflected very clearly the peculiar condition of the English intellectual Establishment. To be a communist, with the declared intention of subverting and destroying the fabric of existing society was to occupy a respectable, and respected position; the difference between a communist and a liberal was merely one of those differences of opinion which arise between the best of friends and which both find mutually stimulating. The underlying assumption was that both shared the same humane and enlightened purpose, and that only questions of method were at issue; so that when, for instance, Stephen Spender wrote a book called *Forward from Liberalism*, it was regarded as perfectly natural that the forward movement should be in the direction of communism. Indeed, the communist in certain respects commanded the admiration, and almost the envy, of the liberal, because he was willing to risk more in the cause to which the liberal was committed; it was almost as if, by a curious inversion of Marxism, the communist in England had come to represent the most advanced and militant section, not of the proletariat, but of the liberal and progressive middle class. And in fact this is in most cases what he did represent, and perhaps this was the final reason for the failure and eventual disruption of the entire left-wing intellectual movement of the 1930s.

To apostasize from communism, on the other hand, was not merely to reject the cause of the proletarian revolution; it was to reject also the progressive purposes which the liberal shared with the communist and which he felt, rather vaguely, that the proletariat might one day help him to realize. And somehow it also besmirched the image which the communist had succeeded in imposing on his liberal collaborators as a man of superior moral integrity, as the fighter who is always in the front line, unhampered by the bourgeois inhibitions and reservations by which the liberal was afflicted.

Thus it was felt that when Guy reneged on communism he did not merely betray his own cause; he disgraced the whole of liberal England and he was ostracized not merely by his comrades in the Party but by most of his friends outside it. He was a man who had fallen from grace, and to some people this was welcome because they felt that he was, in any case, graceless. Various explanations were offered for his conduct, and in the atmosphere of moral indignation which it inspired, not many of them were to his credit. Some said that Guy's sexual life had become so promiscuous as to become a scandal and an offence to the Party which, after all, had long ago abandoned the ideas of sexual morality preached by Lunarcharsky and Madame Kollontai. Communists said that Guy was, after all, a product of Eton and Trinity, and very conscious of it, spent his leisure hours in the company of the gilded intellectuals of Trinity and Kings, and of writers, artists and bourgeois intellectuals, and had failed to bridge the abyss which divided him from the proletariat. He had simply fallen a victim to the seductions of capitalism, and this view seemed to gain in probability when it was rumoured that on leaving Cambridge he had become some kind of political adviser to the House of Rothschild. This particular rumour seemed on the face of it improbable, indeed so bizarre that it introduced into Guy's career an element of farce which was to become increasingly prominent as the years went by.

Guy himself, it was reported, said that he had discovered fundamental errors not so much in the theory as in the practice of communism. The Marxist analysis remained true, but it had been misapplied and the Communist party had become a reactionary movement. The progressive forces were in fact on the extreme Right; he had in fact become, so it was said, some strange new kind of Marxist fascist.

I myself had no opportunity to test the truth of these reports. They came to me from afar, and simply made me feel that Guy had suffered some inexplicable change which had transformed him into an entirely different person from the one I knew. In any case, I was not greatly interested. In 1933, convinced once more that everything that was important in the world was taking place outside England, I had left the *Manchester Guardian* and gone abroad, first to Vienna and then to Berlin, where I had every opportunity of watching the progressive forces of the Right in action. I played at conspiracy with the decimated and demoralized remnants of the German Communist and Social-Democratic parties and talked to storm troopers who were already envisaging a "second revolution" against Hitler; they gave the impression of a country in which all the progressive forces had been ground ruthlessly to pieces under an iron heel. When, on my return to England, I met Guy by accident in St. James's Square I was not in a very receptive frame of mind to listen to a lecture on his new combination of Marxism and fascism. Nevertheless, I accompanied him to a pub near by and I asked him to explain what it was that had so changed his political views. I told him that I thought they were abominable and that he reminded me of those instant converts to fascism in Germany, the *Märzhaase*, who had jumped on Hitler's bandwagon and earned even the contempt of Dr Goebbels.

I was offensive; I was aggressive; I wanted to quarrel. But he took my rudeness calmly and said that communist colonial policy, especially in regard to India, had convinced him of the incompetence and futility of the Party and the Comintern. Their policy was aimed at revolution and the immediate withdrawal of the British from India; yet the objective interest of the Indian masses required that the British should remain until they had completed their historic tasks there. Only then would revolution become a possibility; the only alternative was that India should fall to pieces and relapse into feudalism. But if communist policy was directed at revolution in India, and to a British withdrawal as a necessary preliminary to it, so also was the policy of the British Labour party, though on different and doctrinaire grounds of national self-determination; so also, though on different grounds, was that of the large majority of the Conservative party, which no longer had the courage to undertake responsibility for India; "Men like Irwin," Guy said with contempt; "they're *always* in favour of surrender, on principle, in any circumstances. They don't believe anything's worth fighting for except the Church of England." Guy's contempt for Lord Irwin continued when he became Lord Halifax. Years later he quoted to me with approval a comment on him which he attributed to Churchill: "Halifax has only one principle—grovel, grovel, grovel . . . !"

The only people, said Guy, who really believed in holding India, and had the will to do so, was the Right of the Conservative party, led by Mr Churchill; but the Right was too weak to achieve anything in Britain, where neither the working classes nor the middle classes had any conception of imperial interests which, at the existing stage of capitalist development, were identical with the interests of the colonial peoples. Their only hope of success was in alliance with the extreme Right in Europe, as represented by the German National Socialists and the Italian Fascists, who had no objection to a strengthening of British rule in India so long as they were given a free hand in Europe and the opportunity to expand eastward against the Soviet Union. "But surely that would mean war?" I said, rather stupidly; in those days, we always said it would mean war whenever we objected· to any particular policy.

One must imagine two young men, in the year 1935, sitting in a pub off Pall Mall, drinking, by this time, double whiskies and gravely discussing the fate of the British Empire. It was an absurd enough position, but at the time it was being repeated, in all its absurdity, in some form or other wherever two young men of our particular type of intelligence or folly happened to meet; politics obsessed us as sex and drugs obsess the young today, and sent us on hallucinatory trips like those produced by LSD. I am sure that anyone reading this today will find it very hard to take Guy's arguments seriously; even at the time I did not, and by now I know, as I did not then, that they were invented in order to provide an intellectual defence for a change in his way of life which he had made for quite other and more practical reasons.

Yet considered in themselves they had a kind of mad logic which carried a certain degree of conviction, or could at least be imagined to carry a certain degree of conviction to anyone who was accustomed to Marxist methods of argument and analysis. They were a kind of Marxism-in-the-Looking Glass. And they also carried, in respect to India, overtones of the kind of argument which the Mensheviks had directed against the Bolsheviks in respect to Russia, and more sinister overtones of the arguments by which the German communists had convinced themselves that their greatest enemy was Social Democracy. It was as if Guy, like a deep-sea diver, had plunged into the great ocean of communist dialectics and come up with weapons which would enable him to demonstrate the precise opposite of what he had previously believed and now professed to deny. To me it was a slightly bewildering operation, and yet it had a certain fascination, which was all the greater because his argument was adorned with long disquisitions on the historical role of the British in India, and on the significance of Mr Baldwin and Lord Halifax as traitors who were destined to lead the British Empire to destruction.

The truth is that Guy, in his sober moments, had a power of historical generalization which is one of the rarest intellectual faculties, and which gave conversation with him on political subjects a unique charm and fascination. It was a power which was, I think, completely native and instinctive to him. It might have made him a great historian; instead it made him a communist. He saw historical events as following rational and intelligible principles and as developing according to general laws, and when he talked about politics he demonstrated these laws and principles in action. Somehow this seemed to endow politics with a gravity and dignity which they do not possess when they are regarded merely as a more or less fortuitous series of conflicts between individual wills and ambitions.

My philosophy tutor at Oxford used to tell me that the will is reason acting. It is an absurd definition and not for a moment did I believe it to be true, yet often when arguing with him I had the feeling that it would be far better, for myself and everyone else, if it were. Talking about politics with Guy had something of the same effect on me. He would have said that history was a rational process which we can understand if we wish to and he had the gift of demonstrating this process at work in different historical periods, in different historical events, in certain works of art. I was never able absolutely to believe that these demonstrations, however fascinating, were true; they seemed so often to lead to conclusions which required one to ignore or deny what was going on beneath one's nose. But when I listened to Guy I always felt how much better it would be if his view of history were true than if it were not, and how much more interesting and satisfactory life would be if one knew it was the product of reason and not of chance, whether benevolent or malevolent; how much better one would oneself be if one were oneself a product of reason!

Perhaps Guy's powers of generalization were never more effective than on that day when he was trying to persuade me, for reasons which were thoroughly disreputable and unscrupulous, to accept conclusions in which he did not himself believe. He was so far successful that my bad temper began to vanish, my liking of him began to revive, and I found myself quite willing to listen to his account of what he had been doing to put his conclusions to practical effect. He had become, it seemed, secretary to a member of Parliament who was so far to the right of the Conservative party that it was quite reasonable to call him a fascist. He also shared Guy's sexual tastes, and Guy's duties combined those of giving political advice and assisting him to satisfy his emotional needs. They had, it appeared, recently made a visit to the Rhineland, where a Hitlerjugend camp had fulfilled their ideals both of politics and of love.

Guy talked about his employer with a kind of genial

contempt; he was once again playing his Figaro role of the servant who is really the master, and in describing their Rhineland visit he knew just how to introduce that element of farce which made it absurd rather than distasteful. When he wished, and when he thought it worthwhile, he had an acute insight into people's character and knew exactly how to pander to them; he knew that the best way to please me was to make me laugh, and that day, as we consumed further whiskies, he certainly succeeded. His account of his Rhineland visit, and its extension to the Danube and Budapest, became an immense comic epic, a kind of Nibelungenlied turned into farce; its hero, sailing like Siegfried down the Rhine, was Guy's employer, his head bemused by the servant's elaborately sophisticated defence of fascism and by romantic illusions about German youth which reflected his own more primitive political ideas. Their journey down the Rhine and Danube was interrupted by strange characters who popped up as if from nowhere, like the Anglican Archdeacon much interested in the affairs of the Orthodox Church, whom Guy claimed to have rescued from a particularly scandalous predicament in Vienna. The story was like one of those eighteenth-century picaresque novels in which one is conducted scene by scene through the criminal world, only in this case that underworld was exclusively homosexual and thereby seemed to acquire a specifically modern flavour.

Was it all, or any of it true? There were incidents, dates, events, persons which seemed to verify it; yet its general character was that of a work of imagination rather than a record of fact. Guy's master undoubtedly existed, and he was certainly an MP, with the tastes which Guy ascribed to him and made use of for his own purposes; whether the Archdeacon ever did, or whether he suffered the absurd mishaps which Guy described, I never knew, and yet in later years I was to hear Guy talk of him to others as if there could be no doubt of his existence and the scandalous incidents of his pastoral visit to Budapest were a matter of historical record.

I suppose that, on this occasion, Guy succeeded in amusing me so much that I no longer condemned him quite so wholeheartedly for his conversion to fascism. And I was fascinated by the vivid glimpse he gave me of a homosexual European half-world which I knew would be forever closed to me, even if, as I seriously doubted, it had any existence outside Guy's imagination. And yet, amused as I was by our meeting, I nevertheless had no desire to see him any more; dimly and obscurely I felt that something had happened to him which henceforth made any kind of frankness or sincerity between us impossible. If I had been asked what that feeling was based on I should not have been able to say. I should probably have said that it was due to his political *volte-face*. But at the back of my mind there was the sense that the element of farce in Guy's life had become completely uncontrollable, and that it represented something which was false within, just as some malignant growth may be the symptom of an obscure and profound disturbance of a person's metabolism.

III

In fact, I did not see him again for about a year, which for me was a particularly unhappy one. For a large part of it I was out of a job. I had resigned the research fellowship I had been given at All Souls and rarely went to the college. I had quarrelled with the girl I was supposed to be going to marry and this meant quarrelling with the friends we had in common. For some months I worked on *The Times*, which was not a very satisfactory experience for either of us. Altogether, I felt a failure and tried to keep out of the way of my former friends; in any case, I was too hard up to keep up with their standard of life. I was in fact very lonely and miserable.

But one day I decided to visit the college again, and in the queue at Paddington station found myself standing next to Guy. He was looking remarkably fresh and spruce; his smile, his curly hair, were as boyish and engaging as ever. He told me he was going to visit some friends in the country, a painter who was married to a particularly beautiful and gifted woman; I envied his gift for acquiring talented and interesting friends and thought how much I should like to be doing just what he was doing. We parted on the platform; I spent a rather unhappy weekend at Oxford and on Monday returned to the flat which I had taken in Ebury Street.

I was surprised when, that evening, I entered the pub on the corner of the street and found Guy standing at the bar. I was also pleased, because I spent so many evenings alone at that time that I dreaded the prospect of yet another one; I was all the more pleased because Guy was once again the charming and amusing companion he had been when I first met him.

He talked about his weekend in the country and what wonderful people his hosts were, especially the wife who, by his account, possessed every beauty, every virtue and every talent which are possible in a woman. "You really ought to get to know her," he said. "She's just the girl for you. After all, you're not homosexual; she's rather wasted on me." It was just as if he was making me an offer of her; he was in his Figaro rôle of the go-between, who is all things to all men, and always has something in hand to satisfy every need. I thought rather sadly that there wasn't much in me at that moment which could possibly interest such an exceptional woman; and at the same time I thought how very characteristic it was of Guy to attribute to his friends every possible virtue and charm.

I asked him about his political views, and for a moment he seemed slightly embarrassed, but then he cheerfully refused to discuss the subject, rather like a schoolboy who had committed some peccadillo of which he felt ashamed. But he had given up his post as secretary to the member of Parliament ("He really was *too* absurd") and was now, it seems, acting as a correspondent for various newspapers, though what they were I did not discover. His work took him abroad a great deal; he spoke vaguely of trips to Paris, and as always he seemed to have plenty of money. It appeared also that he had made up the quarrels with his Cambridge friends which had followed his defection from the Communist party. He spoke much, and with profound, almost exaggerated, admiration of some of them who, even though they might not be communists, had still more not been fascists and had deplored Guy's invention of a Marxist version of fascism. It even seemed that he had abandoned it himself.

I spent a very agreeable and interesting evening with him. We drank a great deal, and I was pleased to discover that he lived just round the corner from me in Chester Square. From then on I saw him constantly, and certainly a week hardly ever passed without our meeting. It was indeed only as a result of such repeated meetings that it was borne in upon me what a fantastic pattern his life followed. The trouble was that as one became aware of the pattern, so also one became used to it, and therefore took it for granted. But when one thinks of it in retrospect, and therefore sees it whole, one finds it hard to believe that such a person as Guy ever existed; it is as if he were some gigantic hoax that life had played on one. It is true, of course, that with hindsight many of the bizarre twists and turns in the pattern of his life become intelligible, in a way that they were not then. The curious thing is that the easier it becomes to understand certain details of the pattern which puzzled one then, the more extraordinary the pattern itself becomes.

How well I remember, for instance, walking round to his flat one fine Sunday morning in summer. It was decorated in red, white, and blue, a colour scheme which he claimed was the only one which any reasonable man could ever live with; white walls, blue curtains, red carpet. But this patriotic *décor* was completely submerged in the indescribable debris and confusion of the party which had evidently taken place the night before. Guy himself was in bed, in his blue sheets beneath his red counterpane, which was littered with the Sunday newspapers. On one side of his bed stood a pile of books, including *Middlemarch*, which he must have been reading for the twentieth time, *Martin Chuzzlewit*, Lady Gwendolen Cecil's *Life of Lord Salisbury*, Morley's *Gladstone*, and John Dos Passos's *Manhattan Transfer*. These were all favourite books of his, which he read and re-read continuously, and always with the gift of discovering something new in them at each re-reading.

On the other side of the bed stood two bottles of red wine, a glass, and a very large, very heavy iron saucepan filled to the brim with a kind of thick, grey gruel, compounded of porridge, kippers, bacon, garlic, onion and anything else that may have been lying about in his kitchen. This unappetizing mess he had cooked for himself the previous day, and on it he proposed to subsist until Monday morning. As he pointed out, it was economical, sustaining, and entirely eliminated the problem of cooking for the entire weekend; as for intellectual nourishment, what more could one require than the Sunday newspapers, including the *News of the World*, and the books that were piled up beside him?

So there, for a blissful twenty-four hours, he would lie, at intervals eating his gruel and drinking his wine, while around him moved the ghosts of Lord Salisbury and Mr Pecksniff and Lulu Harcourt. I sat beside him on his bed and we drank one of his bottles of wine while he explained to me precisely why Lord Salisbury had come to back the wrong horse in his foreign policy, and why Mr Pecksniff tells us everything we need to know about Victorian morality; and then I left him and as the day drew on, and the sunshine faded, I felt a slight shiver at the thought of him in his flat high above the square, happy, at peace, with his gruel and his ghosts, as if he were a very particular kind of lunatic in a very particular lunatic asylum of his own.

At about this time my own life took a slight turn for the better, as in 1935 I was made assistant editor of the *Spectator*, for which I was paid £500 a year for three days' work a week and was paid, in addition, for reviewing any books I chose. This was a considerable improvement in my affairs, and I also fell in love with a girl with whom, all that summer, I was very happy. She had a sharp, almost microscopic, painter's eye and was continually making me see things which otherwise I would have missed, so that when one was with her, in the park, in the streets, in the Zoo, one always came home with a collection of *choses vues*, like the hard brightly coloured objects which a magpie picks up for his nest. Her own flat was rather like just such a nest, filled with odd pieces of bric-à-brac that had taken her fancy, with paintings and

drawings given her by her friends and cut-outs from
magazines, and her own bright sharp eye and high clear
voice had something which reminded one of a bird. It
was with her, one Sunday, that I went down to Southampton Water to spend the day on a friend's yacht and there
met Donald Maclean, a young man whom I did not like
and thought rather superior, and whom I was only
interested in because Guy had talked about him with
admiration and had claimed to have gone to bed with him
at Cambridge.

I think I would have been totally happy that year, if it
had not been for the shadow of politics which fell
increasingly heavily upon anyone who took any interest
in such subjects. I had enough money, my job left me a
good deal of leisure, I was in love, and I was writing a
novel. But also the Germans had occupied the Rhineland,
in Germany the concentration camps were full, in 1936
the Spanish Civil War began and several friends of mine
joined the International Brigade and some were killed.
Very often in the evenings I would visit Guy's flat or he
would come to mine and we would drink a bottle of Irish
whiskey and we would discuss for hours what was happening in Europe.

In such discussions I became aware that Guy's political
opinions had undergone yet another transformation. He
no longer talked of the natural alliance between British
conservatives and German fascists. He was now, as I was,
for the Republic in Spain, he was for the Franco-Soviet
pact, he was for the Popular Front. And yet the arguments
he used for such policies had nothing to do with those
which came so easily to me and others like me, which
were based primarily on instinct and emotion, even though
we might try to give them a show of reason. Guy's
arguments had nothing to do with emotion. They were

based on complicated and somewhat cynical analyses of power relationships in Europe, only now they seemed to lead him to very different conclusions from those he had previously arrived at. And he seemed positively to dislike and despise the liberal and humanitarian instincts which led others to the same conclusions as himself.

But since we were now in agreement, had formed as it were a personal Popular Front of our own, it made friendship firmer, even though I sometimes suspected that we made an odd pair of allies and that somehow there was a profound misunderstanding involved in our agreement. When I, for instance, became indignant about the German dive-bombing attacks on defenceless peasants in Spain he would reply coldly that such things were inevitable in a war, and, if it were worth fighting at all, such disasters must be taken for granted; nothing was gained by becoming emotional about them. And when George Orwell and others returned from Spain with somewhat disconcerting reports of the behaviour of the Spanish Republic's Russian allies, he dismissed them as the sob-stories of sentimentalists who willed the end without willing the means and were in effect sabotaging the Republican cause. He was an awkward person to have in agreement with one; so often it turned out that one had agreed about something quite different from what one had intended.

Usually we were alone when we met. I was greatly taken up with my girl, and he with his own sexual adventures, but on occasions when we were both free we made a habit of spending the evening together. Sometimes, however, though much more rarely, he would ask me round to his flat when he had friends there, and at such times it used to strike me forcefully what a very strange collection were gathered in one room together.

There was, for instance, a grossly obese Central European whom I never knew by any other name than Ignatz, who was said to have been a colleague of Bela Kun's in Budapest and to be a correspondent of *Imprecor*, the journal of the Comintern. There was a clever young English historian, who had a kind of pupil-and-master relationship with Guy, from whom he imbibed the principles of the economic interpretation of history. There was a working-class ex-chorus boy called Jimmy, who for a time lived with Guy in his flat as a kind of servant-valet and was later handed round among his friends. There was a mysterious Englishman who conducted some kind of sales agency in the Balkans and came to visit Guy whenever he was in England. There was an anti-Nazi diplomat from the German Embassy. There was a peculiarly detestable Frenchman, named Pfeiffer, who seemed to me to smell of every kind of corruption and later, to my astonishment, suddenly emerged from what I had assumed to be an indecent obscurity as *Chef du Cabinet* to the Prime Minister of France, Edouard Daladier. There was Kim Philby, a young Cambridge friend of Guy's, of whom he always spoke in terms of admiration so excessive that I found it difficult to understand on what objective virtues it was based.

Any or all of these, or others who added even greater oddity to the company, might be found at Guy's flat. I used to wonder what common quality held them, or rather us, together, for after all I was also among them. It could have been said, perhaps, that all were to some degree infected by Marxism, which is a particularly insidious drug to which many unlikely people become addicts. But this was only true about some of them; it was certainly not true, for instance, about the historian, who was by nature and instinct a scholar, even a pedant, and it was even less true about Jimmy and the horrible Pfeiffer, to whom nothing was important except boys and money. It might be said also that the bond was homosexual; but to this again there were exceptions, including myself. In this respect I often felt that I was a fish out of water and indeed that Guy's other friends slightly resented his friendship with so normal a person as myself; the *petit noyau* which Guy had gathered around him had, I felt, certain inner secrets from which I was excluded, and I was not particularly anxious to be initiated into them.

The truth was, I think, that the only real link between the members of Guy's little group was the personality of Guy himself, just as Mme Verdurin's was of her own *petit noyau*. Yet it was not easy to explain his domination over them. Ignatz, for instance, was not an easy person to influence; he was tough, and cynical, and experienced in a much rougher world than most of us had ever seen. And Pfeiffer was the kind of man who would not normally respond to anything except the grossest kind of appeal to self-interest. But none of those men could quite resist the spell which Guy cast on them. It was based partly on genuine intellectual qualities, on his gift for producing original ideas which in his presence seemed extraordinarily fruitful and illuminating but in his absence seemed to wither and fade; they required the force of his personality to make them come alive. Partly it was based on his talent for adapting his own interests to the varying tastes of his friends; for talking about boys to Pfeiffer, about the underworld of politics to Ignatz, about the seventeenth century to the historian, about Dickens to me. But added to all this was the gift of extravagant flattery. Guy seemed to have learned at an early age what most people only accept after long experience; that the thicker flattery is laid on the more palatable it is, for after all, when the recipient has made every reduction from it on the score that it is flattery, there is still left over a substratum of what he can regard as the irreducible truth.

It used to amuse me to observe Guy's power of manipulating his friends, and it was clear to me that on the whole they were chosen precisely because they were willing victims of it. Nor was there any reason to be anything more than amused by it, as by yet another addition to the general spectacle of the human comedy. It would have been absurd that there could be anything serious in the influence of one who was so obviously an anomaly in the social system, so compulsive a drunkard, so completely promiscuous in his sexual life, whose fingernails were so neurotically bitten and filthy, and whose ordinary behaviour was so outrageously and childishly designed to *épater les bourgeois*. One might as well have taken Mme Verdurin seriously. Yet even so, it was, to me at least, an interesting fact that Guy's influence on his friends was never relaxed; secretly, persistently, it was always there, whether they acknowledged it or not.

And indeed he was the most persistent person in achieving his own ends that I have ever known. If one went to the cinema with him and wanted to see Greta Garbo, while Guy wanted to see the Marx Brothers (and he invariably did want to see the Marx Brothers), it was always the Marx Brothers whom one saw. If one went for a drive in his car, and wanted to go to the country while he wanted to go to the seaside, somehow one always found oneself at the seaside. If one wanted to drink white wine and he wanted to drink red (and he always did want to drink red), it was always red wine that one drank. He was persistent as a child is persistent, who always knows it will have its own way if it is willing to behave badly enough; and Guy always was willing to behave badly enough. And in this persistence there lay a formidable power of the will, which, because of the general disorder and absurdity of his personal life, for the most part went unnoticed.

IV

At about this time, I wrote a long review in the *Spectator* of a rather emotional and sentimental book about the condition of the depressed areas; it made the rather simple point that the depressed areas were not an isolated phenomenon but were the result of historical conditions which could not be changed except by concerted political action. I thought it was a good review, but Guy praised it in terms which even I thought exaggerated, as if I had suddenly written a masterpiece; he analysed it at great length, showed me that it contained ideas of a scope and interest which I had never suspected, and generally made me feel that I was a writer of great originality and power. This was unusual, because normally Guy regarded my writing simply as a harmless hobby, or a useful means of earning my living, but not possibly of any wider interest.

One evening, when we were sitting in my flat, with as usual a bottle of John Jameson's whiskey on the table between us, he once again began talking about my review, in the same terms of exaggerated respect. Dimly I felt that I was being made a fool of, and also that praise of such a kind quite obliterated any real merits the review might have had. Slightly irritated, I said to him: "I do think it was a good review, but all the same I don't quite see that it was everything you say it was."

Guy paused for a moment and said: "It shows that you have the heart of the matter in you." There was a note of

134

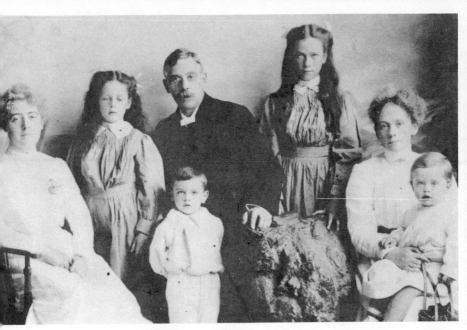

The author, with his father, mother, and family: Aberystwyth 1911. The author is on his mother's knee.

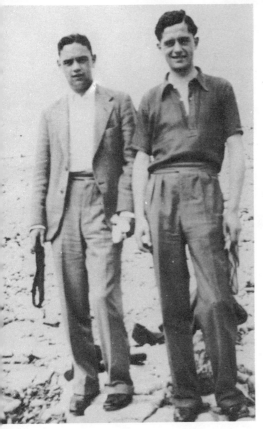

The author *(on the right)* with his brother: ~~1916.~~ 1926 ?

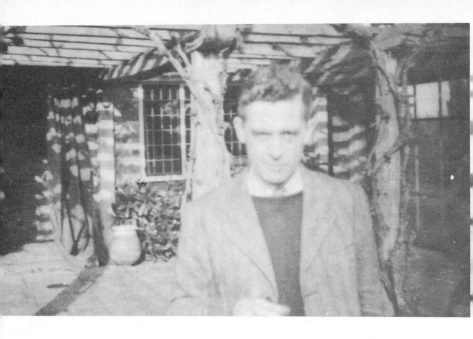

The author: 1930

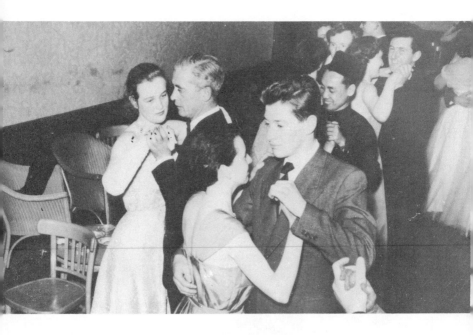

Social occasion at Aberystwyth.

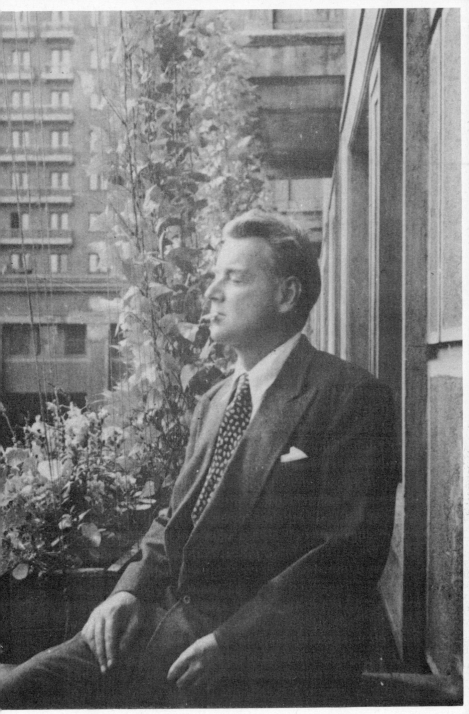

Guy Burgess on the balcony of his Moscow flat. *(Popperfoto)*

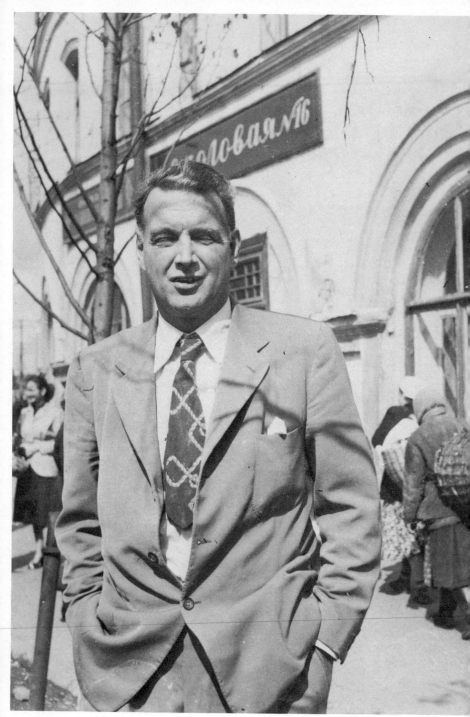

Guy Burgess in Russia, 1956. *(London Express)*

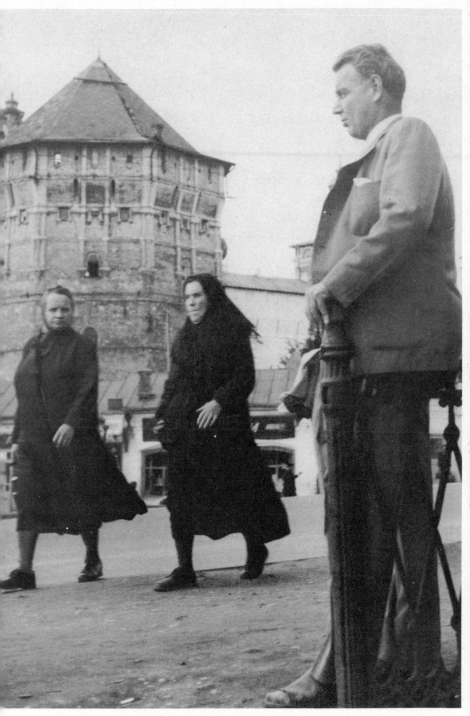

Guy Burgess in Moscow. *(Popperfoto)*

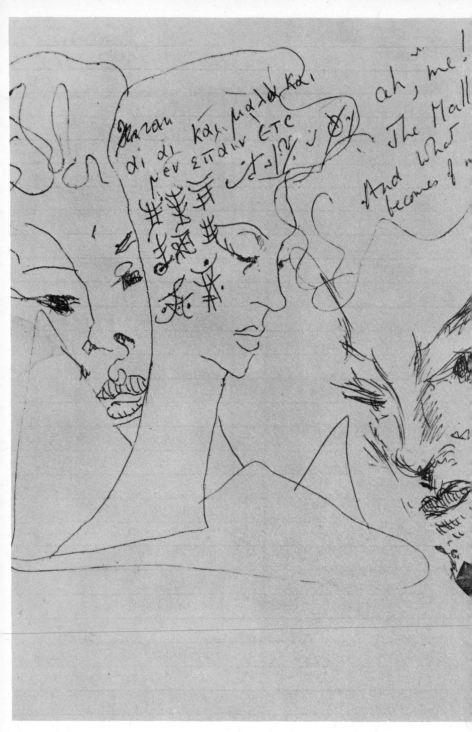

A Burgess drawing.

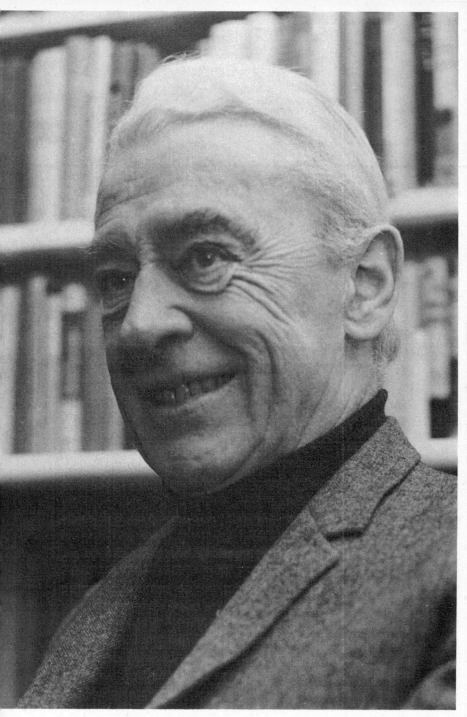
The author. *(Topix)*

solemnity in his voice which surprised me, and besides, I could not attach any meaning at all to his words. The heart of what matter?

"What on earth do you mean?" I said. A strangely detached expression came over his face, as if for the moment I did not exist and his eyes were turned inwards upon some secret known only to himself.

There is in St. Beuve's *Port Royal* a description of how M. de St. Cyran, before giving spiritual direction to a penitent, fell into a profound silence, as if he were waiting for some inner voice to tell him what to say. He must have looked very much as Guy looked to me at that moment. Abstracted, his eyes oddly empty and expressionless, he looked as if he were considering some immensely important decision, with a seriousness and gravity which were so unusual in him that I began to feel uneasy; it was as if I were seeing an entirely different Guy from the one I had known.

Then suddenly the life returned to Guy's eyes and he said, with the same serious expression: "There's something I ought to tell you."

I almost felt relieved. I thought I was going to hear some confession about his personal life or perhaps some more than usually scandalous misdemeanour, though I could not quite see what this could have to do with what had gone before.

"What is it?" I said.

"I want to tell you," he said slowly, "that I am a Comintern agent and have been ever since I came down from Cambridge."

I was so surprised that for a moment the words seemed to convey nothing at all to me, and I had to recover myself while I tried to realize their significance. I saw that Guy was watching me with a steady, intent gaze, which after a moment gave place to a look of—what was it? I found it difficult to say, because it so strangely combined expectation and apprehension.

Then I recovered myself sufficiently to say: "It's not true."

"Why not?" said Guy. Suddenly he seemed brisk and alert.

"I just don't believe you."

"Why not?" he said again. "Why else do you think I've behaved as I have since I left Cambridge? Why should I have left Cambridge at all? Why should I have left the Party and pretended to become a fascist? I hope you didn't believe all that ridiculous rigmarole about India and the conservatives and the Nazis; but I had to invent something to say. They told me that before going underground I must break off all connection with the party as publicly and dramatically as possible, and with anyone connected with it, and try to start a new career of some kind. So I did it. And all that nonsense worked. Do you know, there were some people who not only thought I believed in it myself, but actually thought that it was true. There is really no limit to how stupid people can be."

"But why are you telling me all this?" I said. "What has it got to do with me?"

He gave me a long look, at once challenging and appraising, then said: "I want you to work with me, to help me."

"How can I help you? There's nothing I can do for you."

"Never mind that. You can leave that to us. The question is, will you do it?"

"I don't know," I said. "What could I possibly do to help you?"

"The first thing you'll have to learn is not to ask

questions," he said. "If you're willing to help, you can leave it to me to tell you what to do."

"Does anyone else know about this?" I asked.

He was silent for a moment and subjected me again to a long scrutinizing gaze, as if he were trying to come to a decision.

"A few," he said. "You don't know most of them, and there's every reason why you shouldn't know. But I'll give you one name, so long as you don't ask for any more."

I don't suppose he could have named a person who could have carried more weight with me. He was someone whom I both liked and respected greatly, and with whom I would gladly have joined in any enterprise. Nor was I alone in my admiration; there was no one I knew who did not praise his intelligence, his uprightness, his integrity. Indeed, he quite conspicuously possessed all those virtues which Guy did not; all they had in common, except friendship, was that both were homosexuals. But it now appeared that they were both also Comintern agents.

"But you must never speak to him about it," Guy said. I was so surprised and bewildered that he seemed to be speaking as if from some great distance. "I shouldn't really have mentioned his name to you. It's essential, in this kind of work, that as few people as possible should know who is involved. You must promise never to mention the subject to him."

So I promised, and after that Guy did not speak again that evening either about his work or about the part which he appeared to assume that I would play in it. But he did talk at great length of the anguish it had cost him to break with the Communist party and his friends at Cambridge, of how much he had wished to continue working for a fellowship, of what it had meant to him to be despised and denounced by those whom he liked and admired most and how much he envied those open communists who were not condemned to a life of concealment and subterfuge. His account of the sacrifice he had made for his convictions seemed to me both sincere and painful, and it also seemed to me that perhaps the strain of it might do much to explain the extraordinary aberrations and excesses of his private life.

When I awoke the next morning, my first thought was to remember our conversation of the previous evening, and, as if the day then breaking was a very special one after which nothing would be the same again, I tried to acclimatize myself to the extraordinary fact that a friend of mine was an agent of the Comintern. It is perhaps not necessary to explain that the fact did not shock me; in any case, it would take too long, as it would entail writing the history of an entire generation, and also describing once again the appalling political tragedy of the thirties. I was indeed not shocked; rather, Guy's revelation seemed to provide a genuine and solid basis for my liking and admiration of him, as one who had in the most real sense sacrificed his personal life for what he believed in and, unlike myself, who was merely a political dilettante, had committed himself seriously, professionally, and totally to the tasks of politics, however painful, even repellent, they might be.

The only trouble was that, with Guy about, I could not quite believe it. For after all, what evidence did I have for it except Guy's word, which was notoriously untrustworthy and unreliable. And if it were true that the strain of life as a Comintern agent, the necessity for concealment, for lies, for pretences, might provide an explanation of the tension under which he lived, revealing itself in such orgiastic excesses of drink and sex, might it not equally be true that the story was a fabrication, a mere dream-release and wish-fulfillment of a kind to which he was in any case addicted?

It was hard to see Guy as a hero; easy to see him as a *fantaisiste*. For if his story were true, why should he after all reveal this highly compromising piece of knowledge to me, who as far as I could see could be of no possible help to him and for whom he appeared to have, for the moment at least, no useful employment? Might not Guy's story be one more of his elaborate manœuvres for exercising power over his friends, in this particular case me, for whom it had precisely the romantic quality to which I was most vulnerable? In all Guy's comments on history and politics, illuminating though they often were, or in his accounts of his own adventures, there was a myth-making element which belonged to art rather than sober empirical fact; did not this have precisely the same quality? Did it not provoke in one precisely that willing suspension of disbelief which would endow Guy, in my eyes, with all the romantic virtues of a revolutionary and conspirator, while he himself suffered none of their penalties?

There was of course that one person whose name Guy had revealed to me under so strict an oath of secrecy, who could put all my doubts at rest. But if it were true, as Guy said, that conspiratorial principles demanded that members of an espionage network should have no direct contact with each other, why had he revealed the name to me at all, for under the circumstances it was entirely unnecessary? Except, of course, Guy realized that no other name would have more effect on me in establishing his *bona fides*, as it were, as a Comintern agent.

When I thought about Guy's confession, I felt as if I were trying to solve one of those Chinese puzzles in which one box opens only to reveal another, and not one finally gives up its secret. And just as one box leads one

on to open another, so curiosity drove me on to examine
one possibility after another, because, never having
accepted any statement of Guy's as the plain and un-
qualified truth, I could not now simply take his word for
it that he was what he said he was. The whole thing was
too preposterous, and Guy was too preposterous also.
Yet somehow, at the same time, I also believed he had
been telling the truth.

v

And now it was 1937, and events in Europe began to
move very fast towards the disaster which had threatened
for so long. That summer I attended a conference of the
Writers' International in Paris. The Writers' International was one of the many front organizations which
proliferated from the mind of Willi Müenzenberg as a
means of prosecuting the war against fascism, and
though it included writers of every variety of political
opinion, it was dominated by communists. I was therefore
very surprised when Guy said that he would like to come
to Paris with me. Why should a Comintern agent, who
had advertised so loudly his breach with communism,
associate himself in any way with an openly Left Wing
organization, which he himself must have known to be
a communist front; more especially because the conference
took place under circumstances of considerable publicity.

But one of Guy's most striking characteristics was a
devouring curiosity. He really did not like to think that
anything was ever happening anywhere in which he was
not in some way involved. And he always liked to think,
or pretend, that behind every public event that was
reported in the news there was a private and usually
disreputable story of which he alone knew the secret. It
was as if, in reality or in his own imagination, he was

always searching for the human vices and weaknesses which might explain any public event and which he might one day have an opportunity to exploit. The Writers' International, which oddly enough had a social as well as a political *cachet*, attracted him as a candle attracts the moth.

Guy attended several meetings of the conference with me and was extremely outspoken in his contempt for most of the writers who attended it; his contempt extended both to their literary talents and to their political activities, which he regarded as those of well-meaning but muddleheaded amateurs, and in his comments on them there was always the slightly sinister implication that if, in their flirtations with communism, they really understood what they were doing, they would very quickly think better of it.

The only writer at the conference whom he wholeheartedly admired was Theodore Dreiser, then an old man, white-haired, tall and shambling, with the appearance of a middle-western farmer. He addressed the conference at immense length, and unlike most of the speakers, who devoted themselves chiefly to denouncing the evils of National Socialism, or the wickedness of non-intervention in Spain, or appeals for the consolidation of the Popular Front against fascism (subjects indeed on which few of them were qualified to speak) Dreiser confined himself to a dispassionate and yet extremely moving account of the growth of American capitalism as he had known it during his lifetime, and of the society which had given birth to *Sister Carrie*, *An American Tragedy* and *The Titan*. His address, delivered in his slow, ponderous, American voice, that seemed to reproduce the leaden rhythms of his own prose, plainly bored his audience, because indeed it seemed to have little relevance to the immediate problems of Europe and little of that impassioned revolutionary oratory which came so easily to most of the speakers. It was typical of Guy that it should have inspired him to raptures, for the capitalist system was what passionately interested him, what he understood, what indeed in a strange way he admired. He had for it the same *Hassliebe* as Dreiser had. It was not for love of a new Utopian world that he had become a communist; it was because he thought that capitalism was at the end of its tether and could no longer fulfil its historic mission. He felt that it had betrayed him; in Dreiser's attack on American capitalism, through which there breathed a deep nostalgia for an America that had vanished long ago, he saw the counterpart of his own rejection of British capitalism which could no longer serve the interests of the British people and could no longer shoulder the burdens of Empire. His hatred of capitalism was not that of the idealist who condemns it for its sins; it was that of a disappointed and embittered Imperialist who rejects it because of its failures. Perhaps for that reason it was all the more profound.

It was equally typical of him that, because first Britain, then the United States, had led the world in the development of capitalism, he regarded them as the only countries which in the long run were of any importance. He had an instinctive dislike, even contempt, for other than Anglo-Saxon countries. He did not speak their languages or read their literature and he regarded their politics as childish; in this respect he combined all the prejudices of an American WASP and an English country gentleman, and was as provincial, as insular, in a sense as patriotic, as a reactionary colonel.

This became evident when one evening he and I dined in the Bois de Boulogne with Dreiser and Louis

Aragon. Aragon was brilliant, cultivated, socially *chic*, as only a French communist intellectual can be. He had been converted to communism by way of surrealism, and he looked on communism as the natural heir of all the *avant garde* movements in which he had played a part. Fundamentally, he was less interested in changing the world than in shocking it. No-one could have been less like him than the slightly uncouth, slow moving, slow speaking Dreiser, who beneath his Marxism remained an un-reconstructed Middle Western populist. Both he and Guy were irritated by the intellectual acrobatics which Aragon performed for our benefit. Like two Anglo-Saxon puritans they regarded him as frivolous and affected and superficial; they thought him too clever by half. Their revenge came when he mistakenly entered on a disquisition on English literature, in which his taste was no more sure than that of any other Frenchman. Then they flung themselves upon him with great Anglo-Saxon swings and uppercuts which he as nimbly avoided, until at length he was borne down by the sheer weight of their attack and Guy was given the opportunity to launch into his favourite dissertation on George Eliot as the greatest of English novelists, which was new to them though far from new to me; yet in its way it was so good that I was always glad to listen to it again.

But what, I thought, is a Comintern agent doing in this *galère*, delivering Marxist literary lectures at the top of his voice to two well-known communist writers, from whom he differed only in his greater fidelity to the party line? What had been the point of the elaborate cover he had built up for himself, at so much personal sacrifice, if he could abandon it all so lightheartedly? The puzzle seemed to me all the greater the next morning when Guy went gaily off to see the ineffable Pfeiffer, now Daladier's *homme de confiance*. I was tired of the unending stream of eloquence and rhetoric that flowed through the conference hall and had taken the day off. I waited for him in a *bistro* near the Arc de Triomphe, and when he returned from his meeting he was bubbling over with gaiety and enthusiasm and excitement, as if a few hours' talk with that truly disgusting man were the most delightful experience in the world. It began to seem to me that there was no end to the contradictions in Guy's character, as if I were in contact with an acute case of schizophrenia.

That morning he told me a good deal of backstage political gossip, punctuated by a considerable amount of sexual scandal, and went into some detail about Pfeiffer's secret relations, on Daladier's behalf, with the French Right, together with some hair-raising stories about Pfeiffer's activities as an important officer of the French Boy Scout movement. Some of his stories amused me greatly; but their general effect was to depress me, as they would have depressed anyone who had faith in France as an ally against fascism, for the kind of world they reflected was one whose rottenness had become irremediable. They certainly gave a better picture of the French internal situation at the time than anything which could have been found in the British press, which still regarded France as Britain's strongest and most trust-worthy ally; and Guy's confident prediction that in a crisis France would not fulfil her obligations proved to be perfectly accurate. But none of his information could in any way be described as secret; it was the kind of information which was accessible to any persistent and inquisitive enquirer who would take the trouble to cultivate some of the more seedy and disreputable characters on the French political scene. This was a part which Guy was singularly well equipped to play, and

Pfeiffer was undoubtedly a valuable source. I myself assumed that Guy was exploiting him in his self-confessed rôle as an agent; yet I had to admit to myself that he might just as well have been doing so for some obscure personal motive of his own, or even simply to satisfy his insatiable curiosity.

When we returned home, I did indeed ask him how he disposed of whatever information he obtained. He was annoyed by my question, but he finally said that he made contact with a Russian at regular intervals in a café in the East End. Apart from this, I do not think that he ever again offered any information about his activities as an agent. I formed the impression that if in fact they existed, he regretted having revealed them to me, or that, if they did not, he was annoyed with himself for having made them up.

Perhaps, I thought, it had all been a dream. Perhaps we had been drunk. Perhaps it had been a misunderstanding. And indeed at this time Guy's life seemed to have acquired a certain degree of stability and respectability, so far as such words ever could apply to him, which somehow seemed to make it more unlikely than ever that he was in fact what he had professed to be, an agent of the Comintern. He continued to drink to excess, he still picked up boys at every opportunity, I still used to meet in his flat those oddly ambiguous characters who seemed to live on the criminal fringes of European society. But somehow a certain tension seemed to have disappeared from his life. He had taken a job in the Talks Department of the B.B.C. which he enjoyed very much, and had been given charge of a programme called *This Week in Parliament* which brought him into contact with a great many Members of Parliament who spoke on his programme. This was the kind of thing which Guy liked; I was told both by members of the B.B.C. staff and by Members of Parliament who had talked for him that he did his job very well; so well indeed that to his great amusement he became much sought after, and much wined and dined, by ambitious Members of Parliament anxious to make a name for themselves on his programme. He had an intuitive grasp of the possibilities of broadcasting, and a natural gift for the spoken, as opposed to the written word. He took infinite trouble with his performers' scripts, which were often either dull or incoherent; he was fertile in suggesting ideas to people who often had no ideas of their own, and he could make them sound, on the air, natural, easy and unaffected when by nature they were pompous, or dogmatic or shy.

The truth was that he was genuinely interested in what he was doing, and whenever he was interested in anything he did it well. And it was natural that, in doing so, he should have gained the affection of those who appeared on his programme. They appreciated the trouble that he took, and were gratified when their talks were a success. Radio, not television, was then the way to becoming a 'personality' and I have heard several Members of Parliament who later rose to high office say that they were grateful to Guy and owed to the talks they had given for him their first real start in public life. I have no doubt that some of them, under his influence, found themselves expressing ideas which they had never previously dreamed that they possessed. But at least they were interesting ideas, and people listened to them. On the whole it could be said that for the first time in his life Guy was performing a useful function and performing it very well.

Yet from time to time incidents occurred for which on the whole I could offer no explanation except that he continued to play his professed part as a secret agent. The time of Munich was approaching, and Konrad Henlein, the leader of the Sudeten Deutsch National Socialists in Czechoslovakia, paid a visit to London to establish relations with British political figures who rightly or wrongly he thought might prove useful to his cause. He stayed at the Ebury Hotel, and to my surprise I learned that the boy Jimmy whom I used to meet in Guy's flat had managed to establish himself as the telephone operator at the hotel and at the end of each day delivered to Guy a record of the calls made by and to Henlein, and of the telephone conversations that had taken place. Guy told me of this coup with a kind of schoolboy glee, and yet with the implication that this was part of his espionage activities. I did not question the implication, and yet could not help wondering whether it was not yet another example of his almost megalomaniac compulsion to meddle in matters that were none of his business. And there were hurried and mysterious visits to Paris, and bundles of bank-notes which one suddenly caught sight of stuffed away in his indescribably untidy cupboards, and a general air of conspiratorial activity which had the flavour more of a spy story in a children's magazine than what I imagined to be the sober and discreet methods of an efficient espionage network. The trouble was that I simply could not take Guy seriously in the character of a spy.

Meanwhile, Munich itself occurred; and throughout the crisis Guy, on the basis of what he claimed to be direct information from Pfeiffer, maintained an absolute assurance that there was no conceivable possibility of war, that under no imaginable circumstances would France fight while Daladier was in power, that the British Government was well aware of this, and that consequently we had not the slightest intention of fighting either. In the circumstances of the time, when people were confused, frightened, despairing, Guy's calm assumption of knowledge irritated me considerably and I was perhaps even more irritated when he, and Pfeiffer, proved to be right.

Throughout 1938 and 1939, as war became more and more certain, he maintained this calm assurance, as if he possessed some secret source of information which would prove him right when everyone else was wrong. My own feelings, however, had led me, in 1939, to join the 90th Field Regiment, a Territorial unit stationed in Bloomsbury, conveniently near my office at the *Spectator*. After all, I had spent a large part of the previous two years in trying to persuade people, so far as I could, that it was imperative to resist the advance of National Socialism, by fighting if necessary, and since the time seemed to have come when we would finally have to, I thought I ought to accept the consequences. Guy, of course, like most of my friends, regarded this as simply a foolish and romantic gesture, perhaps even worse, for to many it seemed an act of treachery to fight for any government as detestable as Mr Chamberlain's, and all that it represented. To me it seemed that the time for such refinements was over.

Guy thought me even worse than foolish and romantic, he thought me ludicrous, when in the summer, dressed in my absurd and ill-fitting uniform, ammunition boots clamped to my feet like lead, I went off with my regiment to camp. Ludicrous indeed I felt, because I feel sure that no-one was less well fitted to adopt the profession of arms than I was. And indeed the embrace which the army offered me, submerged for a fortnight in the mud of an artillery camp in the West Country, our guns crawling painfully every day to the mist-veiled hills above, was hardly a warm one. I began to feel very foolish indeed, especially since Guy had gone happily off for a month of sunshine in the South of France. Why, I thought with irritation, did he somehow always manage to get the best of all worlds, and why should I be shivering in the rain and mist of Okehampton while he was hogging it at Antibes? Somehow, there seemed to be no justice in it.

When I returned to my flat in Ebury Street, I stripped off my horrible uniform and flung it into the corner of the room. For one entirely irrational moment, I had the acute pleasure of feeling that at least I should not need it again for another year. But in the next days there came the announcement of the Soviet-German Non-Aggression Pact, and it was clear that war could not be postponed for much longer. The next day, in the evening, Guy appeared in my flat, having driven back from Antibes the moment he had heard the news, left his car at Calais, and crossed over by the night boat. His car was one of the possessions which he valued most in the world, but on this occasion he appeared to have abandoned it without a thought. He was in a state of considerable excitement and exhaustion; but I thought I also noticed something about him which I had never seen before. He was frightened.

He seemed strained and apprehensive in his behaviour towards me, and this was something new in our relations. I imagine he already knew what my feelings would be, and when I denounced the treachery of the Soviet Union and said that the Russians had now made war inevitable, he merely shrugged his shoulders and said calmly that after Munich the Soviet Union was perfectly justified in putting its own security first and indeed that if they had not done so they would have betrayed the interests of the working class both in the Soviet Union and throughout the world. I said that neither he nor the Soviets really understood what Hitler was like, and that one might as well entrust the interests of the working class to a rattlesnake as to him. But he was clearly not interested in my opinions and he spoke wearily, almost absentmindedly, as if he had already discounted this particular argument and wished to get it over as quickly as possible. And indeed it was only when it had come to an inconclusive end, and my indignation had half subsided, that his interest began to revive and the same look of anxiety which I had already observed returned to his face.

"And what do you intend to do?" he said.

"To do? I don't suppose I've any choice. I'll be called up."

"And what about me?" he said. "And the Comintern?"

"I never want to have anything to do with the Comintern for the rest of my life," I said. "Or with you, if you really are one of their agents."

"The best thing to do would be to forget the whole thing," he said.

"I'll be only too glad to forget about it," I said. "After all, it doesn't seem to have any importance now."

"And never mention it again," he said eagerly. "The best thing to do would be to put it out of our minds entirely. As if it had never happened."

"I'll never mention it," I said. "I want to forget about it."

"That's splendid," he said, with obvious relief. "It's exactly what I feel. Now let's go and have a drink."

That was the last drink I had with Guy before the war began. We drank a great deal, as if we both knew that we were drinking the old world out. A few days later I had picked up my uniform from the corner of the room where I had flung it, had rejoined my regiment and found myself in the East India Dock where, unarmed ourselves, we had the slightly absurd task of maintaining order in case of civil disturbance. For the first six months of the war I lived in such a state of complete physical exhaustion that, even if I had wanted to, I could not have devoted any thought to such questions as whether Guy was or was not a spy, or, if he was, whether it was now of any importance at all. All I thought about was such problems as whether one could avoid fatigues in order to snatch a few moments' sleep, or how it was humanly possible to get oneself shaved before presenting oneself on parade by 6 o'clock in the morning. The kind of problem presented by Guy was far too complicated for me to solve or even to contemplate.

VI

War changes all things, materially and morally, and we ourselves change with them. As a private soldier I quite quickly became accustomed to living and behaving in ways which were unlike anything I had ever experienced before, and, not without effort, adapted myself to the code so admirably and succinctly expressed by Brecht: *Erst kommt das Fressen: dann kommt die Moral.* Under the shock of the German-Soviet pact, and its consequence, the war, I had ceased to be a theoretical Marxist, because there was quite obviously something wrong with a doctrine which could lead to, and justify, such results; but I was not far from becoming an unconscious Marxist instead.

War not only changes things; it changes them continuously, as if one found oneself on an endless moving staircase. No sooner had I adjusted myself to life as a gunner than, in the spring of 1940, I was transferred to an Officer Cadet Training Unit at Sandhurst where I struggled to master even more esoteric mysteries of the military life; I found it even harder to be an officer than a private. By the summer I was commanding an infantry platoon in the Royal Welsh Fusiliers, a regiment which seemed hardly to have changed at all since Robert Graves described it in *Goodbye To All That* and David Jones in *In Parenthesis*. In the interval I had managed to write an article for *Horizon*, in reply to an editorial by Cyril Connolly in which he claimed that the only possible attitude for a writer to adopt towards the war was to take as little notice of it as possible; this seemed to me like advising writers to ignore the most profound and all-embracing reality of their time. Guy wrote to tell me that he had liked the article and envied me being a soldier. For the life of me I could not see why he should, nor why he should not be one himself if he wanted to. But at that time in England there was still a feeling that for an intellectual to be a soldier was in some way beneath his dignity and a waste of his talents. To enter the civil service, the Office of Information, the B.B.C., was in some way or another to serve one's country usefully and intelligently, without lending oneself to the more brutal arts of war; but there was something immoral and absurd about being a soldier.

By the end of that year of, for me as for so many others, violent and abrupt transformations of one's personal life I was married, a state I had never hitherto contemplated entering, to a girl I hardly knew and who was hardly out of school; she would not even have known what one was talking about if one had mentioned the word 'Comintern' to her. When I wrote to tell Guy that I was getting married, he replied in a long, affectionate and almost paternal letter about the dangers which both I and my wife were about to incur. I was, he gently but firmly pointed out, an extremely unstable, volatile and undependable character, fickle, changeable, and much addicted to women, who had hitherto shown few signs of being able to support himself, let alone a wife or a family; I was egotistic and pleasure-loving; he could not envisage me as a faithful husband and he hoped I had not deceived my wife into thinking otherwise; in general, it was extremely unwise of me to think of getting married at all and even more foolish and rash of my wife to marry me. In spite of this, he said, if I were really determined to take such a desperate step, he was delighted if I were happy and hoped that we should all three meet at the first possible opportunity.

I showed the letter to my wife, who cried a little, but was quickly reassured when I told her that Guy was only doing, as he thought, his best, by trying to pluck me out of marriage like a brand from the burning; no doubt he thought it would be in both our interests. Even so I could see that she thought it a very odd letter from a very odd person, and suddenly I had a very sharp sense of how very strange a creature Guy must seem when seen through the eyes of someone who had not become as inured to his eccentricities as I had.

His letter, however, also informed me that the opportunity of meeting was not likely to arise soon, as he was leaving England almost immediately for the United States, en route via the Pacific and Vladivostok for the Soviet Union, where he was to join our Embassy staff in Moscow. He told me no more about his mission, nor could I conceive of what possible use he could be in the Soviet Union; I almost felt that he must be indulging his gift for fantasy again, and also had a momentary twinge of apprehension, as of an old toothache, that the fortunes of war should be taking him to Moscow. But in neither case was I seriously worried. War teaches us to accept fantasy as fact, and especially in the first year of the war when everything rigorously followed the rule that it is always the unexpected that happens.

Yet something went wrong with Guy's mission. In a few weeks he was back in England, and when I next met him, in the spring of 1941, he would make no reply to my questions about what happened other than to be even more evasive than usual. Nor would he offer any explanation of a brief paragraph I had read in a newspaper stating that he had been arrested for drunken driving in the Mall and describing him as "a War Office official". The drunken driving he admitted; as to the War Office, he fell impressively silent and said he could tell me nothing because matters of the highest security were involved. Somehow I began to feel that the war and Guy were on a converging course towards a point at which the distinction between fantasy and reality totally disappeared.

In fact, however, I did not see him much during the war; I was occupied with too many other things. But I visited him when on leave in London, and used to talk to him about the war and politics and literature, and envy him because he always seemed to be so much better informed than I was. He now lived in a large and very comfortable flat in Bentinck Street which he shared with a friend from Cambridge days, who by one of those extraordinary metamorphoses which were so common during the war was now a very important member of MI5; and also by two girls who were secretaries in the Ministry of Supply. One of them was gentle, timid and genteel; the other was, in her way, as voracious in her appetites as Guy was in his. Guy used to refer to her as "the Semiramis of Bentinck Street", with a half acknowledged, half suppressed, admiration of her sexual activity. The result was that the flat frequently gave the appearance of a high-class brothel, in which it was impossible to distinguish between the clients, the staff and the management. On the one hand Semiramis entertained a stream of her lovers, including one who, having once entered, "hung up his hat" as Guy said and proved impossible to dislodge. All appeared to be employed in jobs of varying importance, some of the highest, at various ministries; some were communists or ex-communists; all were a fount of gossip about the progress of the war, and the political machine responsible for conducting it, which sometimes amused me, sometimes startled me, and sometimes convinced me that I could not possibly be fighting in the same war as themselves.

On the other hand Guy brought home a series of boys, young men, soldiers, sailors, airmen, whom he had picked up among the thousands who thronged the streets of London at that time; for war, as Proust noticed, provokes an almost tropical flowering of sexual activity behind the lines which is the counterpart of the work of carnage which takes place at the front. The effect was that to spend an evening at Guy's flat was rather like watching a French farce which has been injected with all the elements of a political drama. Bedroom doors opened and shut; strange faces appeared and disappeared down the stairs where they passed some new visitor on his way up; civil servants, politicians, visitors to London, friends and colleagues of Guy's, popped in and out of bed and then continued some absorbing discussion of political intrigue, the progress of the war and the future possibilities of the peace.

I watched this absorbing and animated scene most frequently during 1944, when I had been posted to London to the planning staff of 21 Army Group. I was at that time almost totally immersed in all the details of the invasion; I thought of nothing but beach gradients, underwater obstacles, tables of moon and tide and weather, figures of reinforcements, subversive activity, army-air support, and all the other factors which had to be fitted in precisely to the framework of that immense operation. The work of the planning staff, which for reasons of security was restricted to a minimum, was hard, the hours were long, and an evening at Bentinck Street was like some fantastic entertainment devised specifically to take one's mind off one's labours, though I doubt very much if Field Marshal Montgomery would have greatly approved it. Watching the extraordinary spectacle of life in Bentinck Street, I felt rather like some tired business man who had taken an evening off to visit a strip-tease club.

And yet, an insidious doubt would occasionally creep into my mind. Most of my time in the army had been spent in military intelligence of one kind or another. It is a peculiar, and frequently under-rated, branch of war which induces, in its best practitioners, an almost animal sensitivity to the risks which it involves, not to themselves, but to others. A good military intelligence officer will be continually aware that, by any error or failure on his part, he will be directly responsible for the deaths of many men, in numbers which may vary from those of a platoon to those of an army. In this he is both at an advantage and a disadvantage compared with others engaged in different forms of intelligence operations. In military intelligence you at least know, usually fairly quickly, whether the intelligence you have collected and disseminated has been correct or not; the evidence is before you in the shape of bodies spreadeagled on beaches or on wire, or, quite simply, mangled beyond recognition. I myself, by 1944, had been offered such objective verification; unfortunately for others, it was evidence of my own errors.

The advantage of the military intelligence officer is

that his work, like a scientist's, is subject to empirical proof; his disadvantage, that where he is proved to have been wrong, the evidence is provided by the tortured flesh of men who have been unnecessarily sacrificed, and thus places on his conscience a burden which is hard to bear. In other kinds of intelligence operations, such objective evidence of success or failure is rarely available; one rarely knows whether things have gone well or badly, and indeed one hardly even knows how one would distinguish between the two. On the other hand, this being so, one need never feel that one is directly responsible for whatever results, if any, have been achieved.

I am afraid that the lessons I thought I had learned from my experiences as a military intelligence officer proved useless when I tried to apply them to the case of Guy, simply because the principle of objective verification did not seem to apply. From time to time I used to wonder whether he had been telling me the truth when he said that he was a Comintern agent, and sometimes it even occurred to me that, if indeed he had been telling me the truth, and if he were continuing his activities, the flat in Bentinck Street made an admirable operational base, simply because its exaggerated element of farce would prevent anyone from ever taking it seriously as such. But however much I searched my mind, I could never get any further than totally unverifiable suspicion and speculation, and these, I think rightly, I dismissed.

Certainly Guy himself never directly gave me any reason for thinking that he was anything else than what at the moment he pretended he was, a rather eccentric member of the British intellectual ruling class, who was using the war to advance his own career. Sometimes I used to remember that once, and it seemed already so very long ago, he had asked me to help him in his work as an agent, and it used to amuse me to think that at that moment I happened to be in possession of what I suppose was one of the most valuable, the most important and best kept secrets of the war; this is to say, the exact date, time and place of the invasion of Normandy, the precise naval, military and air force order of battle involved, and the fact that we had misled Stalin about the date at which we intended to launch the operation.

Sometimes, indeed, despite the various *fêtes galantes* which were offered for one's amusement, I used to be irritated almost beyond endurance by the conversation in the flat in Bentinck Street. For those who frequented it, including Guy, were all unconditional partisans of the Soviet Union and completely accepted the scepticism of the Russians, and of the Communist party, with regard to our intention to invade Europe. I used to find it difficult to sit silent while Guy or some visitor asserted on the highest possible authority that the invasion would never take place and that we would never enter Europe until the Russians had rendered any effective resistance impossible.

At length, one day in Spring 1944, I was entrusted with the task of taking the final draft of the operation orders for *Overlord* to each commander-in-chief in turn for his signature. It seemed part of the absurdity that attended any military duty I ever performed that it did not occur to me to take an official car but, with the operation orders in my briefcase, walked out of our head-quarters in St. Paul's and took a taxi. Each commander-in-chief predictably behaved in character. My own, on the authority of his Chief-of-Staff, had already appended his signature. The Naval Commander, Admiral Ramsay, knowing exactly what the Royal Navy had to do and how he proposed to do it, politely asked me where to sign and added his name. The Air Commander, Air Marshal Leigh Mallory, examined every sentence of the long document with the minuteness of a scholar and pedant, and to each of them suggested last minute alterations of phrasing, of style, of punctuation. I had to say that at this moment, after eighteen months of preparation, when at last, in accordance with an infinitely complicated time-table, the men, the ships, the planes were ready to move to their battle stations, no further changes were possible, and somewhat surlily, slowly, painfully, he wrote his name. It was a long and tiring morning, and as I sat in my taxi as we drove from one headquarters to another I could not help wondering what the effect would have been on Guy if I had suddenly ordered it to Bentinck Street and placed *Overlord* in his hands. Would he then, perhaps, have told me what he was up to?

Yet in fact I had by this time dismissed any real suspicions of Guy, even if they sometimes recurred to me as an interesting hypothesis. There were several reasons for this. The first was that even if, before the war, his communist convictions had been strong enough to drive him into the Comintern's espionage network, there was no reason to think that he had not abandoned his underground activities once the war had begun; in this, he would have merely been following the example of so many British communists after the signature of the German-Soviet pact. Secondly, he now took no trouble whatever to conceal his sympathies for the Soviet Union, and this seemed to me a reason for thinking that, whatever else he might be, he was no longer a communist agent. Thirdly, there was the presence in Guy's flat, on terms of the most intimate friendship, of an extremely important member of the security services. I had every reason to believe in his integrity and his intelligence, and at that time he certainly knew more about Guy than I did. He was in a far better position to know about Guy than I was, and if he saw no reason to worry, why should I?

There was yet another reason. Despite the disorder and confusion of Guy's life in Bentinck Street, Guy's career seemed once again to have taken a turn for the better. After his mysterious attachment to the War Office, he had returned to the B.B.C. and from there he had been transferred to the News Department of the Foreign Office. This was a post for which he was admirably adapted. He liked the feeling of having an inside knowledge of British foreign policy and the considerations out of which it emerged. He liked expounding that policy to others, and employing all his ingenuity in showing that British policy was rational and coherent and corresponded to long-term historical interests. He liked and understood journalists, and sympathized with, because he shared, their passion for news, and he enjoyed being on intimate terms with them and exchanging with them that kind of backstage political gossip which was the breath of life to him. All this made him very good at his job, he was evidently very happy in it, and this again made me feel that there was no underlying conflict in his life, such as there would have been if in fact he were pretending to be something quite different from what he was. And once again, if the Foreign Office had no doubts about him, why should I?

Four

WHEN I returned to England from Germany after the war, I had to enter seriously on the business of married life. I now had two small children and before I returned my wife had succeeded in finding a pretty little doll's house in St. John's Wood which, with its garden and its little pillared portico, was as agreeable a place to live in as one could have hoped to discover in bomb-shattered London. And now, perhaps because I was so happily settled in, I began to see more of Guy than at any other period of my life. He liked the domestic atmosphere of my house; he became very fond of my wife and was devoted to the two children, and was an affectionate and generous godfather to the elder of them. He used to compare me to the head of that contented little petit-bourgeois family which made Flaubert exclaim, when he visited them: *Ils sont dans le vrai!* I was not sure that I deserved the compliment, or wholly appreciated it, but to Guy it evidently meant something which was sincerely felt.

Indeed, at this time I began to feel that perhaps some real change had taken place in him. One sign of it was that he had almost entirely ceased to discuss politics with me, almost indeed as if there was no longer anything to discuss. Perhaps this may have been because of the way politics had developed in Britain after the war. The objective of the great anti-Fascist crusade of the 1930s had now been achieved, though in a way, and under circumstances, which no one had foreseen; it almost seemed to have been won in spite, and not because, of the crusaders. But certainly the victory had removed the prime motive for that intense concentration on political issues which had dominated intellectual life in the years before the war. Moreover, the victory of the Labour Party in the election of 1945, and the introduction of the welfare state, had satisfied a large part of the ambitions of the Left and held out the hope of even greater satis-faction; for the intellectual Left there was, for the moment at least, no great cause to fight for.

Guy at least professed to be happy and pleased with Labour's victory, and at the News Department he expounded and justified very ably the ideas and policies which animated the Labour government. After the war indeed, I can remember only three political events which seemed to stimulate him to undertake those long, elaborate and fundamentally hostile analyses of British policy in which he indulged so often before the war. The first was the civil war in Greece, where he was violently opposed to Anglo-American intervention. If one ventured to defend it on the ground that it was the only alternative to a communist dictatorship in Greece, he would sink into a gloomy silence which put an end to any argument. The second event which greatly excited him was the Alger Hiss case in America, to which his reaction was in some ways very odd. From the very first, when the evidence against Hiss was very thin, he professed a firm conviction of his guilt. At dinner in our house one evening a lawyer suggested that in an English court of law Hiss could never have been found guilty. He said that the proceedings against Hiss were a travesty of justice and that he was the victim of a form of persecution which was directed at every manifestation of liberal and progressive thought in the United States. Guy agreed that such a campaign of persecution was in progress. It was, he said, a delayed reaction against Roosevelt and the

New Deal and marked the rise of American fascism in the disguise of anti-communism. But he dismissed the legal arguments against Hiss's conviction as mere pedantry; they showed, he said, how far all lawyers, and especially English ones, lacked any sense of political realities. Hiss was certainly guilty; he was precisely the kind of person who was capable of carrying out the systematic programme of espionage of which Whittaker Chambers, so improbably as it seemed, had accused him; and only a communist could be capable of such a feat. But the implication of what Guy said was that it was Hiss, not Chambers, who deserved our admiration; and indeed he repeated with great relish all those unsavoury rumours which were being used to discredit Chambers in the United States at that time.

The Hiss case fascinated Guy; he saw it as a battle of good and evil in which all the good was on the side of Hiss and all the evil on the side of Chambers. The case fascinated me also; only I saw it in precisely the opposite terms from Guy, for by that time I had come to regard communism, or rather, the Soviet Union in the age of Stalin, as no less an evil, and perhaps an even greater danger, than the Germany of Adolf Hitler. Our divergence of feeling and opinion about Hiss reflected a deeper disagreement which made any form of political discussion increasingly difficult.

The third political event which inspired Guy to eloquence and even passion was the British withdrawal from India, which he denounced as a cowardly betrayal of the Indian masses; he pointed to the partition of India, and the bloodshed by which it was accompanied, as proof that Britain had surrendered her historic mission to maintain the peace and unity of the Indian subcontinent. In such outbursts, there were curious echoes of arguments he had developed during that episode in his life when he had been a supporter of Anglo-German understanding.

Apart from those subjects, Guy refused to discuss politics with me; one reason for this was, as it seemed to me, that it had become impossible to talk about politics at all without discussing, in one context or another, the subjects of communism and the Soviet Union, and Guy was resolutely determined to avoid discussion of either of those matters. If I pressed him on the subject, he simply drank more and faster of whatever he happened to be drinking at the moment, and eventually sank into a kind of morose and alcoholic torpor, hardly speaking a word and, as it seemed, hardly capable of taking in whatever it was one was saying to him.

Such moods became all the more frequent as Guy became more addicted to other forms of drugs, as well as alcohol. He was now perpetually taking sedatives to calm his nerves, and immediately followed them with stimulants in order to counteract their effect; and since he always did everything to excess, he munched whatever tablets he had on hand much as a child will munch its way through a bag of dolly-mixtures until the supply has given out. Combined with a large and steady intake of alcohol, this consumption of drugs, narcotics, sedatives, stimulants, barbiturates, sleeping pills, or *anything*, it seemed, so long as it would modify whatever he happened to be feeling at any particular moment, produced an extraordinary and incalculable alteration of mood, so that one could not possibly tell what condition he would be in from one moment to the next. On the whole, however, it was fair to assume that sooner or later he would lapse into one of those moods of morose silence to which he was more and more frequently liable. And while one could hardly help deploring the extraordinary régime to which he subjected himself, it was also difficult not to be astonished at the equally extraordinary physical vitality which enabled him to survive it. Anyone else, one felt, would have been dead long ago; Guy seemed to suffer no ill effects, except for the recurrent states of silence and profound depression by which he was overcome; one felt sometimes that he was made of some special light alloy, immune to metal fatigue, which was resistant to the normal physical processes of human life.

Those who, like myself, were fond of him, and they were many, would from time to time discuss his moods of depression and wonder whether there was anything that could be done about them or him. The most charitable explanation of them was that, for whatever reason, he was profoundly unhappy and that alcohol and drugs provided him with a kind of oblivion in which he found relief; but this was not a very satisfactory answer, because it only led one to ask why precisely he should be unhappy. There was of course the fact of his being irretrievably homosexual; but certainly Guy was the last person in the world to regard this as a reason for unhappiness.

In my own mind, from time to time, I used to consider two other possible explanations. One was, of course, that he had been telling the truth when, long ago, he had claimed to be a communist agent. It was possible therefore that in the past he had been a spy, and that he continued to be a spy; and that the strain and effort of playing such a part was gradually, slowly but irresistibly proving too much for him. What made one reject such a possibility was, in the first place, the inherent improbability that anyone whom one had known so well for so long was playing such a part; and, secondly, that, apart from that one evening before the war, Guy had never in the slightest way betrayed himself. If the hypothesis were true, it argued a degree of self-control, and a depth of dissimulation, which would be quite extraordinary in anyone, but in Guy seemed entirely out of the question.

There was, however, an alternative possibility which seemed at least equally plausible. This was that Guy may indeed have been a Comintern agent for a short time but had later abandoned his allegiance to communism and was now genuinely trying to create a place for himself in society as it exists in the Western world. But we know very well that such breaks with the past are not accomplished easily; on the ex-communist they inflict profound psychological scars, and painful mental and spiritual lesions, which, in many cases, prevent him from successfully accomplishing the transition from one world to another. Was it not reasonable to suppose that this would be quite sufficient to account for the distressing condition of mind into which Guy had lapsed?

II

So I concluded that, whether or not Guy had once been a spy, he no longer was one. On the whole this seemed to involve far fewer impossibilities than any other view; perhaps I ought to add that it involved the fewest difficulties for myself. It also seemed more likely to be true because at this time Guy, in spite of the extraordinary aberrations in his personal life and behaviour, seemed again to be making what might be called a success of his career, however modestly and even eccentrically. Given his behaviour, one could not quite understand how this could be so; and yet on the whole the facts seemed to show that it was. In 1944 he had transferred from the B.B.C. to the Foreign Office as a temporary press officer; in 1947 he had succeeded in getting himself established, and had become personal secretary to the Minister of State, Hector McNeil. This was a good deal nearer to the heart of the establishment than Guy had previously penetrated, and it even seemed possible that he might now, with a little good luck, be on the verge of a successful career in the foreign service.

MacNeil was not only Guy's superior but a personal friend. He had spoken on Guy's radio programme and the two of them had liked each other, and MacNeil had considerable respect for Guy's political judgement, his fertility in ideas, and his gift for analysing concrete political situations. Indeed, he listened to Guy's views with a deference which often seemed as if it were Guy who was his superior, rather than the other way round; MacNeil felt that Guy had a valuable contribution to make in the foreign service and he tried to foster and advance him in his diplomatic career with an almost paternal care. The truth was that MacNeil was a very nice man, and Guy had managed to find the way into his affections.

Yet I often used to wonder how any Minister could possibly tolerate Guy as a subordinate. He was quite incredibly disorderly and irregular in his habits; he had very little of a civil servant's capacity for expressing himself clearly and briefly on paper; and one imagined that some at least of his personal idiosyncrasies could not fail to be irritating, and even offensive, in a well-regulated office. He was, for instance, inordinately fond of garlic, and was as impregnated by its aroma as a French peasant. He ate it not, like most people, as a herb or a seasoning, but as a vegetable or a fruit; he kept knobs of it in his pockets or in his desk and from time to time gobbled a few of them like apples. He told me one day, with triumph and amusement, that a departmental minute had been

167

circulated to the following effect: "Mr Burgess will in future refrain from eating garlic during office hours." He laughed; I laughed; who could have helped laughing? The minute had just that air of farce which Guy always succeeded in introducing into the most solemn proceedings. But I never noticed that the supplies, or the smell, of garlic ever became any the less.

There was indeed a general air of good-natured disorganization and disorder in the secretaries' room in the Minister of State's office in those days, which to myself, who had a certain awe of the Foreign Office, made it a very surprising, interesting and rather attractive place; certainly it had the charm of being entirely untainted by that air of industry, sobriety and decorum which I have always associated with HM diplomatic service. When I used to call on Guy there, I would normally find him and his colleague, the Private Secretary, facing each other across an enormous desk littered with an assortment of official papers and a large selection of the daily press, of which Guy was a devoted and assiduous student. There would also be a few volumes from the London Library, a few sketches and caricatures which Guy had tossed off in the course of the day (it was one of his talents that he drew extremely well) and a few sets of humorous verse composed by his colleague.

The room had that particular uncared for and dilapidated atmosphere which it is the genius of the British civil service and British Railways to create wherever they penetrate, but to this Guy and his colleague had added a few touches of their own; that is to say, there seemed to be even more overflowing ashtrays, burned-out matches and empty cups of tea than usual, while a few gnawed knobs of garlic, as if mice had been at them, added a bizarre and original element to the disorder. The bare and austere neatness of the normal civil servant's desk had entirely disappeared under a luxurious profusion of papers, documents, files, memoranda that looked as if the entire Foreign Office archives had overflowed into the room. Messengers entered, looked vainly for in- and out-trays under the deluge of paper, and dropped their files and messages wherever Guy indicated with a negligent wave of the hand. Either he or his colleague would pick up one or two of them, marked URGENT, glance at them for a moment with a look of distaste, and as hurriedly restore them to their appointed place among the débris.

In this scene of disorder, Guy and his colleague would sit and discuss the events of the day; or, rather more often, of the night before, for the Private Secretary was, in his own way, as addicted to the *chasse au bonheur* as the Personal Secretary, though his tastes were more normal. Conversation in the secretaries' room was very largely devoted to whatever pleasures they had enjoyed the night before, either together or apart, and to reporting whatever material for gossip or scandal they had picked up in the course of it. Not the Chanceries of the world, but the night clubs and brothels, the pubs and cafés of London, were the objects of their interest and discussion, which from time to time would be interrupted by a buzz from the adjoining room where sat the Minister of State, occupied, I used to imagine, in vainly trying to restore order to the chaos created in his affairs by his two assistants. The peremptory summons would normally be greeted by some such words as:

"Oh Lord, there's Hector again."

"What on earth can HE want?"

"I can't think."

"Perhaps you'd better go in, Guy."

"Oh no! He can't possibly want *me*. I've been in *twice* already today. You go. It's your turn."

After that there would be a silence, while they waited to see if the Minister would ring again. If he did not, it would be agreed that he could not really want anything at all, and that it really was too bad of him to disturb them to no purpose.

All this was a reflection of Guy's basic attitude that established institutions were created for his own convenience and use; he regarded them with a mixture of contempt, indulgence and amusement as if fundamentally they were playthings which only children could take seriously. One evening I called on him to borrow a book he had promised to lend me. This was Kinsey's *Report on the Sexual Activities in the Human Male*, which was as yet unobtainable in England but Guy had been sent from the United States. When I called, he told me there was such a press of would-be borrowers in the Foreign Office that he had been forced to hide it.

"I'll have to go and get it," he said. "Come with me."

I followed him out of the room and down the dusty corridors of the Foreign Office. "I wish they'd have Kinsey in here," he said. "He'd find some pretty queer evidence about the human male." We came to what was evidently a very important room indeed, so that even Guy stood abashed for a moment on its threshold. Then he said:

"It's all right. He's not here," opened the door into a vast room which seemed to be all faded crimson and brocade, with heavy, rather shabby curtains and a carpet that had seen better days. Yet it had a kind of dilapidated grandeur, and I felt alarmed.

"Where are we?" I said. "Whose room is this?"

"It's the Foreign Secretary's. I thought you'd like to see it. Don't you love it? I do."

"For God's sake," I said, "let's get out. I've no business to be in here."

"Oh, it's all right," Guy said, "Ernie's away. Besides, I've got to get Kinsey for you."

At one end of the room there was a bookcase filled with what appeared to be reference books. Guy fumbled among them for a moment, then withdrew his hand holding the Kinsey Report.

"There you are," he said, offering it to me.

"What on earth is it doing here?" I said.

"Oh, I keep it here," he said. "Everyone's trying to get hold of it, and I had to hide it somewhere safe. No one would think of looking for it here and if Ernie found it he wouldn't know what it was about. It couldn't be safer."

Then he showed me a portrait of Lord Salisbury and once again repeated his favourite story that, on his death bed, Lord Salisbury had said he had backed the wrong horse in failing to come to an agreement with Russia. I have never known the origin of this story, and was never quite sure whether Guy had found it in Lady Gwendolen Cecil or whether he had invented it. But Guy always repeated it as if it came from some sacred text to which only he possessed the key. Perhaps the reason was that it seemed to bestow the authority of Lord Salisbury, for whom he had a veneration verging on idolatry, on the policy of friendship and alliance with the Soviet Union, of which he had become a passionate and persuasive advocate.

III

Despite his drink and his drugs, his sudden surrenders to despondency and silence, there were still periods in Guy's life when gaiety predominated, and at such times he was always charming; only such moods became increasingly rarer, and they were almost entirely a matter of the private and not the public life. He had moved into a flat in Bond Street, which he had redecorated in his favourite colour scheme of red-white-and-blue and furnished with those particular articles of furniture which were essential to his scheme of life. First, an enormous double bed with an elaborate Italian ornamental head of stripped oak. Then a gramophone, on which he could interminably play to himself his favourite records. They made a curious collection in which *The Marriage of Figaro* easily came first, but was followed by a song from a pre-war musical by Beverley Nichols:

> *I've got a little white room*
> *With a window by the sea*

and, more recently, by a song of Peter Lind Hayes;

> *The tin roof leaks and the chimney leans,*
> *I've a hole in the seat of my old blue jeans,*
> *And I've ate the last of them pork and beans;*
> *Life gets tedious, don't it.*

It would require an elaborate analysis of Guy's intellectual and emotional processes to show why such works had a common appeal to him; after the war his musical resources had been increased by a small and battered harmonium which he had rescued from a bombed house during the blitz and had carried half way across London on his back. In the evenings, when the noise of the Bond Street traffic had died down, he would seat himself at this precious acquisition and pick out pieces of Mozart and Handel to himself with one finger. After this came his books, a curiously mixed collection of Victorian and American novels, British nineteenth-century history, and a large number of books on Marxism and communism. Lastly, there was a model of a fully rigged frigate in full sail enclosed in a glass bottle, a symbol of his enduring love and admiration for the British Navy.

In these surroundings he could contrive to be happy. Apart from his inordinate consumption of drink and cigarettes, he made very few demands on life, and even his drinking varied and he never drank when he was alone, so that for considerable periods he was comparatively temperate. His only extravagance was motor cars, for which he had a passion which was both aesthetic and historical. He had an exhaustive knowledge of every make and model since the first days of motoring, and would relate each variation in design to the particular historical circumstances in which it had taken place; for the T-model Ford, and for Henry Ford himself, he had an almost religious veneration. They represented for him one of the supreme achievements, and one of the supreme creative geniuses, of an age of social and technical revolution to which political revolution was the natural sequel.

He had an equal and similar passion for the Reform Club, of which he was a devoted member. It had, after all, been built at a period which was for him the culmination of English history, and its architecture, its furniture (and indeed even some of its members) belonged to an age in which, in his eyes, society had been everything that it should be, that is to say, technically and politically progressive and expansive. He was in this sense one of the most old-fashioned of British patriots and, more than anything, it was the sense that Britain had ceased to play the part of a dominant and progressive world power that turned him against her, as if his love had been rejected. Indeed in the days when he still used to discuss communism with me I used sometimes to have the disconcerting feeling that he looked upon the Soviet Union as a kind of reincarnation of Victorian England, only with the irritating difference that it was inhabited by foreigners who did not speak English. And indeed, from this point of view, it was perhaps not altogether inappropriate that he should have ended his life in Moscow, for there he might still have found shabby remnants of vanished splendour, rags and tatters of a vanished imperial age which might almost have made him feel that he was back in the Reform Club ordering one of those immense beakers of port which to the waiters were known as "a double Burgess".

From Bond Street to the Foreign Office; from the Foreign Office to the Reform Club; from the Reform Club to a pub, or a party or a night club; occasional forays into smart society, because he liked to be friends with the great; Guy's life had begun to follow a routine in which even alcoholic or sexual indulgence fitted into a pattern of almost monotonous regularity. It might even seem, at moments, that Guy was growing respectable. He dropped hints that he was thinking of getting married, and once at least he professed to have decided on the bride, though I think that the lady in question would have been surprised and perhaps alarmed to know that she had been selected as Guy's intended victim. There were times also when he spoke of giving up the Foreign Office and finding some other career for himself; for a period he flirted with the idea of becoming the motoring correspondent of *Country Life*. I even began to feel that his interest in politics which, whatever side he professed to be on, had always been intense and even obsessive, had perhaps begun to die altogether, and that now he wished, however hopelessly, to settle down as an ordinary, one can hardly say respectable, but least politically neutral member of society.

174

One day I said to him that he seemed to me to have lost his interest in politics. He said nothing. For some reason this annoyed and irritated me. I had always felt that Guy's political interests, whether misdirected or not, were the most important part of him, and that if they died, the most valuable part of him would die with them; it was as if by abandoning them he was betraying himself.

I said I assumed that he had long ago abandoned his activities as an agent, and asked how in fact they had finally come to an end. Again he made no reply, and when I persisted he first said he refused to discuss the matter with me and then relapsed into sullen silence. This irritated me even more, and even alarmed me; his silence seemed to suggest that in fact Guy really had been a spy and might even continue to be one. I felt that somehow I must at last put an end to the doubts and suspicions which had troubled me for so many years. I was provoked into saying, untruthfully, that I had written a record of our conversation on the subject before the war, and in particular of his declaration to me that he was a Comintern agent, and that for my own protection I had deposited a sealed copy of it with my lawyer.

To my surprise, this startled Guy out of his silence; indeed he showed every symptom of extreme agitation, asked angrily why on earth I had done anything so foolish, begged me to destroy the document and said that if it were ever made public it would not only put an end to his career at the Foreign Office but prevent him from following any other. Indeed, his agitation was so great that I had difficulty in calming him; and I was so disconcerted by the storm my harmless fiction had caused that it did not even occur to me that Guy's alarm was somewhat exaggerated if, as he professed, he was only concerned about his diplomatic career.

When I thought over the incident later, it left me with a sense of uneasiness and disquiet; it seemed to me that somehow Guy's reaction had been out of character and had been quite different from anything I would have expected. There had been real and genuine fear in his face and for a moment it had been as if I was looking at a person I have never seen before. I had not succeeded in putting an end to my suspicions; rather, they had been strengthened to a point at which one conclusion seemed to be unavoidable.

Given Guy's character and behaviour as I had known them before the war, it had been quite reasonable to assume that he had been boasting or romancing when he claimed to be a Comintern agent; it was quite impossible to go on doing so when the mere idea that his statement was on record should throw him into such extreme agitation. If the claim had been invention there was no reason whatever why he should be frightened, for I, certainly, had no evidence whatever to show that it was true. I could only conclude that he had been telling me the truth, that he now greatly regretted telling me, and that at the time he really had been what he claimed to be, an agent of the Comintern. The only question that remained was, had he ever ceased to be one?

IV

The certainty that one of one's greatest friends has been, and may still be, a spy is a considerable shock, even though one has considered such a possibility for a long time. Suspicion is a long way from certainty and when one's affections are concerned one is always inclined to give its object the benefit of the doubt. Certainty, even if it is only subjective, no longer leaves room for such a possibility. Moreover, it leaves one with a very unpleasant problem on one's hands; what, if anything, is one going to do about it?

Merely to ask that question was to be made acutely conscious of the change that had taken place in one's political beliefs since the end of the war. Before 1939, if like thousands of young men one was passionately opposed to the policies of the British Government, and believed that they could only end in war, one was as likely to admire as condemn anyone who had enlisted as an agent of the Comintern; especially because in those days the Comintern still enjoyed a prestige which did not necessarily attach to the Soviet Union. After the Soviet-German pact it became difficult, if not impossible, for anyone except a committed and convinced communist to maintain such an attitude, and after the war it became even more impossible to do so with each year that passed. Even so, it was still difficult to condemn anyone for having held and acted upon political convictions which one had in fact shared; in Guy's case, it seemed to me, it was only possible to condemn his behaviour if, in the very changed circumstances of 1945 and after, he had persisted in underground activities which might have been excusable, and even praiseworthy, during the period of the Spanish Civil War and of Munich.

It was with some relief that I came to the conclusion that this was very unlikely. During the war, Guy had lived on close and intimate terms with people who had occupied extremely responsible positions in the British security services; they were in fact the people who had known him best during that period, and certainly far better than I had. It seemed to me inconceivable that such people were not in a far better position to judge Guy's activities during the war and after than I was. If there was anything in those activities of which the security services should be informed, they were the very people best placed to know. It seemed to me therefore that if anything needed to be done, it had almost certainly been done already; and if nothing had been done, it was not necessary to do anything.

Indeed, on reflection, it seemed to me that the whole pattern of Guy's life after the war confirmed the correctness of this conclusion. As I have said, his career at the Foreign Office, if not brilliant, was at least more successful than might have been expected, and this seemed to show that, if there was anything against him, it was not anything which his superiors took very seriously; certainly nothing so serious as a suspicion that he might constitute a security risk.

There were other aspects of his life which seemed to confirm that his career as a spy had ceased long ago. One of his most striking personal characteristics was his devotion to a small number of friends who had remained his friends through all the vicissitudes of his life. Now, by a curious chain of historical events, some of these had risen to posts of great authority in the security services, and it was precisely these whose company Guy frequented most, with whom he lived on the most intimate and friendly terms, and who were in the best position to know everything about him. Indeed, when I met him in their company, as I sometimes did, he showed so much knowledge of their works that it was clear he was on the most confidential terms with them, and they with him. Frequently, they spoke in a kind of professional shorthand which was completely unintelligible to me.

I think in particular of one small group of people who played a particularly important part in Guy's social life. Guy used to meet them regularly every Monday evening for the particular purpose of attending the music-hall at

the Chelsea Palace in the King's Road; it became part of
the repetitive pattern of his life that every Monday
evening was religiously set aside for this little social
excursion, for which the party was always the same; two
women, Guy, a high official of MI5 and another of MI6.
Even to me, who knew them well, they always used to
seem a strangely constituted quartet. There was something *queer* about them, not in the homosexual sense, but
in the sense which applies to members of the security
services when they are off duty. At the same time, Guy's
relations with them reassured me, because I could not
believe that Guy could be on such peculiarly close terms
with these particular individuals if there was any justification at all for the occasional qualms of doubt and
uneasiness which seized me in respect to him. Indeed, in
such circumstances, to have any doubts at all about him
seemed to open up such appalling prospects that it
seemed best to suppress them. It seemed safer, wiser, and
less presumptuous to assume that since both the Foreign
Office and the security services were perfectly happy about
Guy's *bona fides* there was no reason for anyone else to
question them.

Indeed, during this period Guy's relations with the
security services seemed to become increasingly intimate
and confidential. Of course, the very existence of a secret
service was for Guy a challenge, almost an affront, to his
curiosity. He had always been possessed by a devouring
interest in affairs that were none of his business; he liked
the *coulisses* of politics, and for a Marxist he was curiously
inclined to accept the conspiratorial theory of history. He
liked to know, or pretend to know, what no one else knew,
he liked to surprise one with information about matters
that were no concern of his, derived from sources which
he could not, or would not, reveal; the trouble was that

one could never be sure whether the ultimate source was not his own imagination. Yet, even so, it is certain that, during the period after the war, both in London and later in Washington, Guy amassed a large body of information about the working of the security services and about their officers. It would be easy to exaggerate the amount of strictly political information available to him; a minor Foreign Office official does not have access to many state secrets. But it would be difficult to exaggerate the value to an enemy, or a potential enemy, of the knowledge which he had acquired about the machinery and methods of the security services, their organization, and the names and positions of those who worked in them. It is the kind of information which a rival security service values most, because it is the hardest to obtain, so that as a potential defector Guy's value was very high indeed.

It was yet another symptom of the astonishing and schizophrenic contradictions in his character that he could not keep even this kind of knowledge to himself, and in 1949 his lack of discretion nearly proved fatal to him. He had been for a holiday to North Africa, visiting Gibraltar *en route*, and leaving behind him wherever he went a record of drinking bouts and brawls which would have done credit to a Dimitri Karamazov. He had also at each stage in his travels insisted on visiting the local representatives of MI6 and on discussing their characters, habits, opinions and professional inadequacies with anyone who chose to listen to him in any bar in which he happened to be drinking. In addition, he had personally applied himself to the task of trying to persuade MI6's slightly startled representatives of the errors of British foreign policy in general and the follies of MI6 in particular. His journey through the Maghreb became a kind of wild Odyssey of indiscretions, and it is not surprising that such behaviour on the part of a member of HM Foreign Office should have created some consternation. Not unnaturally, it was reported to London, so that for a moment it seemed that his diplomatic career would come to an abrupt end, and indeed he himself spoke as if he had no alternative but to resign or be dismissed.

On occasions when he was in trouble Guy would often consult me; he did so in a spirit of mingled contrition and amusement, and never failed to recount each disaster as if it were simply one more incident in the gigantic farce of his life, so that it seemed as if it were not so much he as the Comic Muse herself who was responsible. On this occasion he had prepared, for the benefit of the Foreign Office, a memorandum explaining and defending his conduct, which he showed me and asked for my advice. It was not a very impressive document; it was long drawn out, tedious, and extremely detailed and by entering into very complicated and elaborate explanations of incidents which were quite obviously indefensible only seemed to magnify their importance. I felt at the end of it that it made Guy's case even worse than it was at the beginning. So I advised him to reduce the memorandum to the shortest possible compass and to say as little as possible about any of the particular charges against him, reserving the right to ask for a board of enquiry if he were threatened with anything more serious than a reprimand. The manœuvre seemed to work very well and having been in due course severely reprimanded Guy happily and only slightly chastened resumed his diplomatic career.

This incident had the effect of weakening even further any suspicion that still lingered in my mind that Guy might still be an enemy agent. For whatever view one might have held about the efficiency of the NKVD, it seemed quite impossible that any responsible intelligence agency could possibly employ anyone capable of such behaviour; there was in it a kind of infantilism which made one doubt whether he was really capable of serious work. It seemed to imply that by now Guy's irresponsibility had become completely out of control, and indeed at the time there were even grounds for thinking that perhaps some process of mental degeneration was taking place. A short time before he had suffered a severe concussion, as a result of having been pushed down the stairs during a drunken evening spent at *Le Bœuf sur le Toit* in the company of his amiable colleague, the Private Secretary to the Minister of State, and its effects upon him had been alarming. He suffered from severe headaches, his dependence on drugs increased. He obtained his supplies through a boy friend, whose sister was a vet and prescribed for Guy the same dosage as for a horse. Drugs, combined with alcohol made him more or less insensible for considerable periods in which, when he was not silent and morose, his speech was rambling and incoherent. The holiday in North Africa had been intended partly as a rest cure, even though it turned out to be something quite different.

Yet, even so, my doubts were not set entirely at rest. His conduct in Tangier might indeed have been a purely temporary aberration, due to his concussion; it did not necessarily mean that he was no longer capable of carrying out his duties, whatever they might be. As for the argument that no serious organization would contemplate employing him in his mental condition at that time, I could not help reflecting that the Foreign Office seemed quite content to, despite his misdemeanours. So that really one was no further than before.

Later, the Foreign Office in a White Paper said of Guy's behaviour that "while on holiday abroad (he) had been guilty of indiscreet talk about secret matters of which he had official knowledge". This was misleading in several ways. It implied that this was an isolated incident in Guy's life, whereas his behaviour in North Africa was in no significant way different from his behaviour in London, where his indiscretions were equally flagrant. The only difference was that in North Africa people had been surprised by them. The White Paper equally implied that his indiscretions related to matters with which he was officially concerned; in fact, they related to matters with which he had no reason whatever to be concerned and were breaches of information which he had acquired only as a result of his compulsive curiosity, his devouring interest in everything affecting the security services, his obstinate refusal to accept that, in his case, there were any matters which could be regarded as secrets. To him, the very word *secret* was a call to battle, a challenge which he never failed to accept. He hunted out secrets like a hound after truffles.

v

Alas! Guy's African holiday, even though he escaped its severest consequences, was the beginning of the end, or perhaps the end in itself, of what had been, comparatively speaking, a stable and successful period in Guy's career of public service. Under the protective wing of Hector McNeil, who never wavered in his devotion to Guy, he had been to some extent sheltered from the buffetings of fortune, and indeed McNeil showed an almost pathetic paternal interest in his welfare. In 1949, however, McNeil became Secretary of State for Scotland, and his successor as Secretary of State, Mr Kenneth

Younger, perhaps understandably did not take over his two extraordinary secretaries. The Private Secretary was posted to Moscow, the Personal Secretary to the Foreign Office's Far Eastern Department.

The transfer did not improve Guy's position. As secretary to the Minister of State, he had exercised a certain amount of personal influence on the Minister himself, and Guy had taken every advantage of his position. As a Third Secretary in the Far Eastern Department he was merely a very junior and humble member of the diplomatic hierarchy, and his position seemed all the humbler because of his age; at thirty-eight he must have been one of the most elderly Third Secretaries there has ever been. Nevertheless, he made the most of what opportunities the Far Eastern Department offered, more especially as a propagandist for the People's Republic of China; it could even be said that he made himself useful.

His interest in China was an old one, which had begun as far back as the days when he was a communist in Cambridge; he was a particular admirer of the Indian revolutionary, M. N. Roy, who from 1926 to 1927 had been the Comintern's representative in China. Guy had the kind of mind which is extremely tenacious of the knowledge and ideas acquired in youth; in some respects, indeed, he might be said to have never advanced beyond them, but he was extremely able and ingenious in adapting them to changed circumstances. In the Far Eastern Department he made himself useful by producing reasonable, comprehensive and historically based arguments in defence of the British policy of recognizing the Communist government of China, and was adept at expounding and interpreting the Chinese Revolution in terms which career diplomats could understand. In those days, professional theorists of the Chinese Revolution were hard to find, more especially if their theories appeared to coincide with British interests; so much so that when, in the summer of 1949, the Foreign Office held a weekend summer school at Oxford it was Guy who was chosen to lecture Britain's representatives, who included members both of MI5 and MI6, on *Red China*. And no doubt it was because of his renewed interest in the Chinese Revolution, in explaining which Marxist arguments could be so ingeniously used to justify British recognition of the People's Republic, that Guy's virulent anti-Americanism became increasingly acute as the months went by; for after all it was the United States which was the greatest obstacle to the adoption of the kind of policy towards China which in Guy's view Britain should in her own interests adopt.

Guy's genuine interest and belief in the Chinese Revolution were sufficient to keep him happy in the Far Eastern Department; he always came nearest to happiness when his mind was being actively and usefully employed. Unfortunately, he had friends, and particularly Hector McNeil, who were interested in advancing his diplomatic career. During the whole of his service in the Foreign Office, he had been stationed in London; if he were to achieve promotion, it was clear that sooner or later he would have to undertake a tour of duty abroad, and that his appointment in the Far Eastern Department could only be an interlude before he emerged as an accredited representative of Her Majesty's Government on some foreign mission. Guy, however, did not respond to such projects at all sympathetically. For one thing, he was far too fond of London, of his Bond Street flat, of his friends, of the Reform Club; he was far too settled in his own peculiar ways to want to live abroad for any length of time. He regarded England, and London, as the only

place in which a reasonable man could want to live; he
was as convinced as Dr Johnson that there was nowhere
else which could compare with them as a means to
happiness, pleasure or interest. *Abroad* was for him a place
which had only two functions: to provide material for
political theories and diplomatic negotiations, and opportunities for holidays on which one could behave with even
less restraint than at home.

He protested energetically that he had no wish whatever
to be posted abroad; that he had no desire for promotion
and that if he had an ambition it was to return to the
News Department, in which he felt that his particular
abilities could be most usefully employed; in fact, that
he objected strongly to leaving London, even though
this might mean that he never rose above the very
subordinate position which he then occupied.

His protests were in vain. His well wishers, and the
Foreign Office, decided that a move could no longer be
postponed and that Guy should be posted to our Embassy
in Washington. This particular decision was, from every
conceivable point of view, a calamity. Even if there were
any possibility that Guy could be groomed for a normal
diplomatic career, for which foreign service was essential,
there was certainly no foreign mission for which he was
more unsuited than Washington. During the year he
had spent in the Far Eastern Department he had become
increasingly and aggressively anti-American and made
no secret of his belief that the United States was an
urgent menace to peace and was dominated by forces
which were determined to lead her, and Great Britain,
unless she succeeded in disassociating herself, into war
against the Soviet Union. No one who knew Guy could
believe that, in Washington, he was likely to disguise
such beliefs in order to spare the susceptibilities of

Americans; and given also that he was unlikely to make any change in his personal behaviour, it was impossible to contemplate his posting to Washington except with dismay. Sending him to Washington was as appropriate an appointment as if the Americans had sent us Senator Joseph McCarthy as their Ambassador.

Guy had no illusions about his suitability for the post, and if he could possibly have managed to stay in London he would have. We discussed it all one evening shortly before he was due to leave and he did not conceal his gloom at the prospect before him. Nothing I could say would relieve his depression; he spoke of resigning from the Foreign Office, and I could not really understand why he didn't, because I could not see that it held any future for him. Somehow one could not imagine him devoting a lifetime to writing inter-departmental minutes or attending Embassy cocktail parties. But then one could not really see that there was anything which held a future for him.

The prospect seemed all the darker because in the preceding months, for the first time since I had known him, he seemed to have been short of money. It was one of the oddest aspects of his character that, despite all his irresponsibility, his apparent lack of any kind of self control, his gift, which amounted to genius, for involving himself in disaster, in some respects he was extremely punctilious; he never missed an appointment, he was never late, and until shortly before he left for Washington he always lived within his income and never ran into debt. But now he had borrowed quite a large sum from an affluent friend of mine and I knew that he had also borrowed money elsewhere. I was surprised and puzzled by this, because it was so marked a change in a pattern of behaviour that had persisted for so long, and because

I could see no change in his circumstances to account for it.

But much as he disliked the thought of Washington, he had a kind of toughness and resiliency which made him respond to adversity and made one feel that he would surmount this as he had surmounted so many other reverses. He had survived so many setbacks, so many crises, so many appalling incidents that one almost felt that the ordinary rules of human life did not apply to him and that whatever happened to him he would always emerge unscathed.

And he did not leave without suitably celebrating or mourning his departure by giving a party in his flat. I went with an eager sense of curiosity, because Guy very rarely gave parties; when he drank, he liked to drink with at most a few friends, and preferably one, because his friends were so curiously ill-assorted that they did not combine easily; and besides he was apt to tell them so many conflicting stories about himself that if they met there was always the danger that he might be found out. I was curious to see what Guy's friends looked like when they were all collected together and I could not help feeling that we might make a very strange company. But even I was not quite prepared for the curious collection of humanity which had gathered to say goodbye to him. Some were so respectable, like the Secretary of State for Scotland and his successor at the Foreign Office, that they could be regarded as the most authentic pillars of the Establishment; there were others, like three distinguished members of the security services, whose whole lives were devoted to guarding against any attempt to undermine the Establishment either from within or from without. There was a distinguished and homosexual writer of impeccable social origins. There was a member of the German Embassy, also homosexual, who before the war had actively plotted against Hitler and now lives in the German Democratic Republic. There were two women who seemed to be even more out of place than anyone else. There was Jimmy, who so long ago listened in to telephone calls and now lived in Guy's flat and acted as his general factotum. There were two very tough working-class young men, who had very obviously been picked up off the streets either that very evening or not very long before. And the party proceeded as such parties normally do; the Establishment figures gradually departed, drink flowed faster, one of the young men hit another over the head with a bottle, another left with the distinguished writer who woke up in the morning to find his flat stripped of all its valuables.

As the evening wore on, as it were to a predestined conclusion, I could not help wondering what we all thought we were doing there and what a very odd collection we were. The only connection between us was Guy; it might almost have been a malicious joke on his part to bring us all together. And indeed, if one analysed each member of the party's particular relation to Guy, we presented a very strange commentary on English society at that moment. Some of them were friends he had known since they were undergraduates together, and some had been fellow members of his in the Communist party. Some were his professional colleagues in the Foreign Office. Some were there simply to minister to his and each other's physical pleasures; some were spies and hunters of spies; some were present merely because at some time or other they had succumbed to Guy's personality. The elaborate web of inter-relationships which had brought them together included strands which were political, social, personal, erotic, even criminal, enough indeed to supply the material for a whole society. And in some odd way this society was the same society which I had first come to know at Oxford, only with the years it had suffered a mutation which had profoundly changed its character. I remember thinking that the oddest thing of all about the party was that no one seemed to think there was anything odd about it at all.

VI

Under these distinguished auspices Guy departed to America and perhaps the United States never received a stranger guest. It so happened that soon after he left, I and my family moved from London to the country, and the move, combined with Guy's departure, seemed to make a very definite break in my life. Certainly Guy's absence left a distinct void in it, but at the same time it made life a good deal easier. One was no longer liable to be rung up late at night and asked whether he might come round for a drink, or to have him for lunch and find him still with you at breakfast. Most of all, with Guy in America, the entire problem of Guy, like some over-hanging shadow, was removed and one did not have to think about it any longer.

At infrequent intervals I heard from him, one letter an emotional outpouring because the village in which I lived happened to be the one in which his mother and father had spent their honeymoon; others of which the common theme was the increasingly virulent quality of his anti-Americanism. For Senator Joe McCarthy's anti-communist crusade was now in full swing, and Guy had come to the conclusion that he was both the most powerful and the most representative politician in the United States, and that the future of America was in his hands. What aroused Guy almost to hysteria was Senator

McCarthy's identification of communism with homosexuality in the United States, and especially in the State Department. "Things have reached such a pitch", he wrote, "that two members of the State Department daren't dine together in public for fear of being called homosexuals and therefore Communists." It was no use replying that McCarthyism in America was the symptom of a hysteria which would not last for long and that his own reaction to McCarthyism was also an hysterical symptom. This only earned me the stern reproof that I knew nothing about American politics and indeed seemed to have become incapable of understanding politics at all; and he repeated his conviction that McCarthy was the most powerful politician in America who would inevitably and deliberately lead or drive her into a nuclear war.

It was during Guy's absence in America that a slightly bizarre incident brought me once again into contact with Donald Maclean. He was now, after recovering from a nervous breakdown, head of the American Department at the Foreign Office, and his appointment had coincided with Guy's departure for America. I had not seen him for about fifteen years, had heard Guy and a few other friends mention his name once or twice, but otherwise had never had any reason even to think of him. Very soon after his appointment my wife and I and two friends went very late one evening to the Gargoyle Club, which at that time was a favourite resort of intellectuals. Maclean was already there and was very drunk; I would not even have recognized him if I had not been told who he was. To my astonishment he lurched over to my table, addressed me by name, and then said in an extremely aggressive and menacing voice, "I know all about you. You used to be one of us, but you ratted."

I thought for a moment he was going to assault me, as by now he was leaning over the table towards me; at the critical moment, however, drunkenness betrayed him, his legs crumpled beneath him, and he sank slowly to his knees. There he stayed, his hands clutching the edge of the table, his large white face suspended like a moon at about the level of my chest, and from this absurd position he proceeded to direct an incoherent stream of abuse at me, which continued until after a few more moments of denunciation he rose unsteadily to his feet and stumbled away.

My first reaction to this ridiculous scene was rage and irritation, but one of my friends who knew Maclean explained patiently that he was very drunk and frequently was very drunk and that in such a condition he was not really responsible for his actions and therefore I should take no notice. So we left the Gargoyle for another night-club; as we left I could not help wondering whether my contacts with the Foreign Office were at all typical and thought how splendidly Maclean would have fitted into the late Minister of State's office, if only he could have made room for one more lunatic among his secretaries.

The idea made me laugh and my annoyance passed, but when I thought about the incident again I was puzzled. What could Maclean have meant by: *You used to be one of us, but you ratted?* It could only mean, it seemed to me, that he thought that I had once been a communist, as he had been, and was no longer. But I hardly knew Maclean, had not seen him for fifteen years, and there was no reason why he should be any more interested in my political ideas than those of hundreds of young men who had gone through the same process. And why the slightly sinister: *I know all about you*, as if he shared some secret about me which was unknown to the rest of the world? This could not have any reference to my political opinions which, after all, had never been concealed from anyone.

A dreadful suspicion began to dawn upon me that Maclean had been a collaborator of Guy's in his espionage activities and that Guy had told him he had enlisted me also. So far as I could see there could be no other explanation which was at all possible, yet I shrank from accepting it because of the appalling consequences it entailed. It meant that Guy had been telling me the truth about himself; for surely he would not have troubled to tell the same lie to two people, and in particular to Maclean, who by now held a very senior appointment in the Foreign Office? It also meant that Guy had been telling me the truth when he said there were others associated with him in his work, though he had not mentioned Maclean's name.

But two spies in the Foreign Office? It seemed preposterous. But there were even worse conclusions to be drawn. If Guy was a spy, what was I to make of the fact that several of his most intimate friends held important posts in the intelligence service? Was I to assume that he had told them what he told me? It seemed hardly credible. Or was I to assume that he had not? In which case I had also to assume that, as a spy, Guy had successfully deceived them, even though some of them knew him a great deal better than I did; or at least, so I had always believed.

At that time, in 1950, one was a little less ignorant about the Soviet espionage system than one had been in the 1930s. After all, there had been the Hiss case, there had been a number of well-documented books on the subject, there had been the Canadian spy trial which had led to the conviction of Allan Nunn May, who had himself been a friend of Guy's and Maclean's at Cambridge. Even so, I found it impossible to accept the terrible implications of Maclean's drunken outburst, if it meant what I took it to mean. So once again I looked for another explanation. The only one I could find was that, as members of the Communist party while at Cambridge, both Guy and Maclean had been enlisted by the Comintern into their espionage organization. For some time they had acted as Comintern agents; later however they had severed their connections with whatever organization they had worked for, though retaining their communist beliefs, and with time had gradually become more outspoken about them, for the very reason that it was no longer so necessary to conceal them. And holding such beliefs, as I no longer did since the German-Soviet pact and the outbreak of the war, they might well regard me as a political renegade who had deserted to the forces of capitalism and reaction.

It was not an entirely satisfactory explanation, but it had a greater plausibility and credibility than the alternative; certainly it was the only one I could find which allowed me to avoid the conclusion that Guy and Maclean were members of an espionage network which had penetrated the Foreign Office and possibly our intelligence services. As such, with some relief, I accepted it. Guy was, after all, my friend; and besides, I had no ambition to be the British Whittaker Chambers, and even if I had, I had nothing like the mass of evidence which Chambers had at his disposal. I had, at the most, a suspicion, which might prove to be entirely without foundation.

VII

For some time after this, I did not hear from Guy or write to him, and so I did not tell him of my curious encounter with Maclean in the Gargoyle. But from other sources I gathered that things were not going well for him. Visitors to America who had met him in Washington had complained to the Foreign Office about his violent anti-Americanism, and when I finally received a letter from him, which was indeed a scream of rage against American policy, it was clear from his own account that he was not in very good odour at the Embassy. This did not, however, appear to trouble him much; the approval of his superiors was not something by which Guy ever set great store. Moreover, life in Washington was made pleasant for him because he was living with an old Cambridge friend, Kim Philby, who, under the cover of a second secretary at the Embassy, was the representative of MI6 in the United States. My heart bled for Guy's host and even more for his host's wife. I thought of the cigarette ends stuffed down the backs of sofas, the scorched eiderdowns, the iron-willed determination to have garlic in every dish, including porridge and Christmas pudding, the endless drinking, the terrible trail of havoc which Guy left behind him everywhere. Yet I knew his misdemeanours would be readily forgiven, for Guy had a devotion to his friends which inspired an equal and answering devotion, and strangely enough he never quite strained it beyond breaking point; though the strain, admittedly, was often very great indeed.

Somehow I had a feeling, however, that Guy's stay in Washington would not be unduly prolonged; I felt that he could not live his kind of life anywhere except in England, where people had become so accustomed to his conduct and behaviour that they took them for granted and almost ceased to notice how very odd they were. In England he was like some bizarre feature of the landscape, like The Needles or Stonehenge, which local inhabitants have long ceased to notice unless their attention is directed to them; strangers and foreigners did not find it so easy to overlook his eccentricities which, even for an Englishman, were outrageous. So I was not surprised when, in the Spring of 1951, I received a letter from Guy saying that he had once again become involved in one of those unfortunate incidents which were so frequent in his experience. By his own account, he had been driving south from Washington to deliver a lecture at a military academy; I believe the subject was once again *Red China*. On the way, he gave a lift to a young man. The journey was a long one and Guy drove far and, as always, very fast; beginning to feel tired, he asked the young man to take the wheel for a time. He then fell asleep and woke to find that the young man was being arrested for speeding; feeling that he himself was responsible, Guy produced his passport and pleaded diplomatic immunity, which had considerably annoyed the Governor of Virginia, who had made the most energetic protests to the Embassy against Guy's behaviour. The Embassy, understandably, was equally annoyed.

The story had the salient characteristics of most of Guy's stories about himself, that is to say, it covered most of the facts, in particular the fact that he was in trouble once again, while contriving to show that on the whole they were to his credit. Nor was I surprised to receive a further letter saying that he was really in disgrace and was being sent home; he was arriving at Southampton on May 7th and would like to come immediately and stay with me in the country. He added that he would probably have to resign or be dismissed from the foreign service, but that this did not greatly worry him as he already had another job in view which he would like to discuss with me.

I must confess that I looked forward to his arrival with considerable interest, but also with some trepidation. I had been ill and had been told to stay in the country to rest and recuperate, and somehow visits from Guy did not conduce to rest and recuperation. Besides, after nearly a year's absence, one could not foresee what kind of condition he would arrive in. When he did arrive, however, after a night in London, and with his luggage still unpacked, we were all most agreeably surprised. America, despite his troubles, seemed to have been good for him. He looked young and well and was in much better shape physically than when he had left England. He did not munch pills continually, and even drank only in moderation. He was delighted to see my children and had brought them some very handsome and expensive presents from New York. And perhaps because of the higher standards of personal appearance required in the United States, he looked much *cleaner* than when he left, as if the Americans had put him through a special dry-cleaning machine for visiting diplomats. His suit was freshly pressed, his handkerchief was clean, even his fingernails were almost clean; so far as such improbable words could ever be applied to Guy, he was spick-and-span. He was gay and charming and delightful as I had not remembered him for many years, and very excited about our house and appreciative of what we had done with it; he gave us long, scurrilous and extremely amusing accounts of life in Washington, and especially in the Embassy, and we were all delighted to find him in such good order and humour.

But it was also evident that he was labouring under a tremendous sense of excitement, as if he were under intense internal pressures. Soon he began to launch into a fierce indictment of America and American policy and the menace of McCarthyism, the imminence of war and the total inability of our Washington Embassy and the Foreign Office to comprehend the catastrophe with which we were all faced. He had with him a briefcase which he never left out of his sight and said that he had some papers which he wanted to show me; "but first of all", he said, "I must show you this", and with an air of good-natured triumph produced a personal letter of thanks from Mr Anthony Eden (as he was then) for the extremely interesting tour of Washington on which Guy had conducted him on his recent visit to the United States. I had a sudden vision of Guy and the Foreign Secretary standing on the steps of Grant's tomb while Guy analysed in great detail the economic conditions in the United States which had made a hero out of a whiskey-drinking ex-regular officer who had been a failure in civilian life; and why this precise concatenation of circumstances had led to the strategy and victory of Vicksburg, followed I was sure by a convincing demonstration that just as the economic situation of the United States in 1860 had determined the triumph of Grant, so in 1950 it required the triumph of Senator McCarthy. Did Mr Eden enjoy the lecture? Did he even listen? It would have been hard to say; but his letter was very polite and Guy was almost childishly proud of it.

When he had carefully restored it to his pocket, he opened his briefcase and produced a long draft despatch, as from the Embassy in Washington to the Foreign Office. It was an able analysis of the elements in the American political situation, both long term and short term, which in Guy's opinion constituted an immense danger to peace; but it was unbalanced in the sense that it took no account whatever of any counteracting factors. Guy said with some bitterness that his ambassador, Sir

Oliver Franks, had refused to forward the despatch to London, that this was the culmination of a series of reverses he had suffered in trying to make his views effective in Washington, and that these rather than his personal misdemeanours were the reason for his being sent home in disgrace. In all this there was not the slightest awareness that a Third Secretary is not expected to have independent political views and certainly cannot hope that, even if they are brilliant, they are likely to have the official endorsement of his Ambassador. I suddenly had the slightly queasy feeling that I was talking to a lunatic. I had never had quite the same feeling about Guy before, in spite of all the monstrosities of his behaviour. He had always had an extremely sharp insight into the workings of the English social and bureaucratic system. Now he seemed to be throwing all this away, for some purpose which I found myself totally incapable of understanding.

It did not make things any clearer to me when Guy proceeded to say, with the new kind of excitement and agitation which were something quite different from anything I had ever known about him before, that he was not content to leave matters as they were, and that he intended to show his rejected despatch to those people he knew, both within and outside the Foreign Office, who were in any kind of position to influence British foreign policy. I asked him who in particular he meant, and he said that in the first place he would show it to the head of the Far Eastern Department and also to the ex-Minister of State for Foreign Affairs, Kenneth Younger. These, he said, were honest and intelligent men who would understand what he was talking about.

I told him that he was wasting his time and his energy and that, though much of his rejected despatch was a true account of the political situation in the United States, it was not nearly objective enough to persuade people who presumably had other and perhaps better sources of information to change their minds. I was quite suddenly appalled by realizing how extraordinarily abstract, and for that reason unrealistic, Guy's views about politics were. My comment for a moment depressed him, but that evening nothing could really affect his good humour and his happiness at being back in England. For a moment they gave me a sad and acute feeling of what a marvellous human being he might have been under better and happier circumstances.

To all my criticisms of his draft he replied, with a kind of cheerful stoicism, that I didn't really understand about politics, or the enormous issues that were at stake, and that there was not much point in discussing them with me. We went on to gossip about Washington and what had happened in England during his absence; he remained cheerful and charming, yet I had the sense that his mind was not really on what we were saying and that the inner tension within him was only awaiting a more sympathetic audience to express itself more completely.

It was a very beautiful spring evening. After dinner we walked down to the river and went to the village pub where we drank beer and Guy told me about his plans for the future. He said he had been suspended from duty and it was extremely unlikely that he would be reinstated. Yet he was extremely optimistic about himself, because through the influence of an old Etonian friend he had received the offer of an appointment as diplomatic correspondent to a leading national newspaper. He seemed to look forward to the job with pleasure and anticipation, though with some twinges of conscience because, as he said, the paper's conservative views were not exactly his own. I tried to reassure him by saying that there was no reason why a correspondent should share his paper's political views, and said that after so many years of working for bureaucratic organizations like the B.B.C. and the Foreign Office it would be good for him to enjoy the relatively independent life of a journalist; and after all, if what he wanted to do was to bring about a change in British foreign policy, he couldn't do better than to start in his own paper. He laughed, and said I might be right, but I had a feeling that he wasn't really listening to me and that his mind was elsewhere. As we walked home from the pub he said very seriously that he was very sorry about my illness, hoped I would soon get better, and that it wasn't really fair to bother me with his own personal problems at such a time; it would be better, he said, if we avoided political discussions because by now our views obviously lay so far apart that it would only lead to argument. I suddenly had the feeling that in some sense he was counting me out and writing me off as a person who could be of any help to him, and that he had decided it would be a waste of time, or worse, to talk to me about many of the things he wished to discuss. In some kind of way it was like coming to the end of a long journey.

In the morning he got up very early and went down to the river and then came back and played for a long time with the children. Since my wife and I were still in bed, he asked the cook to give him his breakfast and later she said what a charming guest he had been and how beautifully he had played with the children, and the children said what fun it had been to have him to stay and when would he come again. When at length I managed to get up, we went up together on the train to London. In the train he gossiped and chattered placidly and amiably and again I had the impression that, despite his obsessions about American foreign policy, he was physically and mentally in much better condition than before he went to Washington. In London we went into a pub and arranged that he should come and spend the following weekend with me; he seemed almost childishly pleased at the prospect of doing so. While we were in the pub a friend of mine came in who also knew Guy and we gossiped for a few moments and then Guy left. I watched Guy's broad-shouldered figure, bent slightly forward like a bear's, and with a bear's heavy gait, as he went through the swing doors of the pub. It was the last time I ever saw him. When he had gone, my friend remarked how much better Guy was in looks and appearance since he had been in Washington, and how much good America seemed to have done him.

"So clean! So *spruce*!" he kept on muttering in surprise.

VIII

Oddly enough, as the weekend approached, I felt that I did not want to hear any more of Guy's anti-American ravings; they annoyed and depressed me, and yet they seemed the only thing that really engaged his interest or feeling. Since there was really no hurry to see him again, and there would be plenty of further opportunities, I thought it might perhaps be just as well to postpone his visit; there were times when a visit from Guy could seem oppressive and exhausting, as if his shadow blacked out everything else. I telephoned him and asked if he would mind my putting him off. He cheerfully assented and said he would come to see me again soon. I asked him what he had done about his memorandum, and he said that the only person he had as yet shown it to was Donald Maclean. I was surprised, because Maclean had not been mentioned among those to whom he had intended to show it. He also said that he was pursuing negotiations about his appointment as a diplomatic correspondent and was going to dine with his prospective editor the following week. There was nothing in his voice or manner during the conversation to indicate that he was in any way disturbed or distressed; rather, he seemed more than usually cheerful and happy.

So I did not see him at the weekend of the following week, and if I thought of him at all it was to assume that he was actually engaged in trying to reorganize his life. Later, I received accounts of his behaviour from friends of his which I found very difficult to reconcile with the impression I had formed of him. It appeared that he had relapsed into drinking heavily and taking large quantities of drugs and pills of various descriptions. Also a young American, whom Guy had picked up on the boat coming back from America, had suddenly made an appearance and had apparently inspired a series of emotional storms and crises in which both Guy and some of his friends were involved.

On the Thursday night, May 24th, of that week I went to All Souls. I had become Estates Bursar of the college and the time had come for me to prepare my terminal report on the college's finances to its stated general meeting. On the Saturday morning my wife telephoned me, and asked whether Guy had come to Oxford to see me. I was surprised. Why should he have? So I said no, and asked what made her think he might have come. She said she had received a telephone call from Jimmy, the young man who shared Guy's flat, and that he was evidently in a great state of agitation. It appeared that Guy had not returned to the flat on Friday night and that Jimmy seemed to be extremely alarmed by his absence. He had said that Guy had never before done such a thing without letting him know, though, as my wife said, Guy had in fact often enough spent a night with us without telling anyone. She said that Jimmy seemed rather hysterical about the whole matter without very much reason, and I agreed with her; hysteria had come to seem to me an almost inevitable function of all homosexual relationships. There were, after all, all kinds of reasons which would account for Guy's absence from home for one night; he might have got drunk and ended up in a variety of unlikely places, or he might simply have stayed the night in a friend's flat as he had so often done with us.

Yet my wife also seemed slightly distressed and puzzled. She said that on Friday morning Guy had telephoned her, and that they had had a long conversation, only it had been so incoherent and so little of it had made any sense to her that she had assumed he was either drunk or under the influence of drugs and had not really paid much attention to what he was saying. I told her not to be worried, that Jimmy was almost certainly being hysterical, and that really the world had become a very strange place if a person like Guy couldn't spend a night away from home without causing a panic. Yet I am not sure that even at that moment some slight premonition of disaster did not cross my mind; all the same, I assumed that Guy had simply been on a spree or bender of some kind and thought no more about the matter until I returned home on Sunday evening. I began to become seriously alarmed when my wife recounted to me the substance of her telephone conversation with Guy the previous Friday.

He had telephoned her from the Reform Club, and it was her he wished to talk to, not to me. The conversation had lasted for about twenty minutes and my wife said it was difficult to give a coherent account of it because Guy had sounded so strange that she really hardly understood what he was saying. Among other things, he had said that he was about to do something which would surprise and shock many people but he was sure it was the right thing to do. My wife, trying to attach some meaning to these mysterious words, thought he was talking about his prospective job as a diplomatic correspondent and meant that some people would think it dishonest of him to join a paper whose political views were so much at variance with his own. But she did not take such qualms of conscience very seriously and uttered the kind of soothing words one uses to drunkards or babies, and said there really was no reason for him to be so distressed. Guy had gone on to say that he would not see me for some time and that this was really for the best, because we no longer saw eye to eye politically; he realized that I was ill and if we met we were bound to disagree and this would only distress me. But I would understand what he was going to do, and indeed was the only one of his friends who would; he repeated this several times with great insistence and then repeated that we should not see each other for some time, perhaps a very long time. By now my wife had resigned herself to a conversation which seemed to her entirely incomprehensible, and confined herself to uttering appropriate words as Guy continued incoherently to repeat that he knew he was doing the right thing and that I would understand.

I should add here that I had never told my wife, or indeed anyone else except one other person, of my conversation with Guy before the war in which he had said he was a Comintern agent; even though I had so often wondered and speculated about it, I had regarded it as a thing of the past which was better forgotten. So it is not surprising that she could not have made much sense out of Guy's message. And from her account of it, it was not easy for me to make out very clearly what Guy meant. But at least I made this out: that the message was a warning of some kind, and also a farewell. I was not sure what the warning was, but at least it meant that Guy was going away and that this involved some action which might be regarded as sensational even for Guy. I did not by any means think quite so consecutively, but having got so far I suddenly had an absolutely sure and certain, if irrational, intuition that Guy had gone to the Soviet Union.

I may say that in the weeks and months that followed I was never quite so certain of this again; but for a moment the confusion created by all the inconsistencies and aberrations of Guy's behaviour seemed to disappear, and the explanation seemed to be crystal clear. So much so that to my wife's utter bewilderment, and almost without thinking, I said: "He's gone to Moscow." Yet even as I spoke the words I felt how wildly improbable and fantastic they would sound to anyone else, and I had only to look at my wife's face to see that this was so. Indeed, when once we began to discuss Guy's absence and to consider all the other and far more plausible reasons why Guy should have gone away for a few days, the more improbable my initial conjecture became.

Yet, after so many years of doubt and speculation, I felt that this time it really was not for me to decide what was the truth of the matter, even though anything I did was likely to involve me in ridicule or perhaps worse. If I was right about what Guy had done, then it seemed to me that even the claims of friendship did not allow me to be silent any more, because the consequences of his action might be in innumerable ways disastrous. I had no choice, I felt, except to inform the proper authorities of Guy's absence, and of what I thought to be the reason for it, even though I didn't much look forward to the polite incredulity with which my story was likely to be received. I explained to my wife what I thought I should do and my reasons for doing it, and even then felt how very odd my explanation sounded, even to a sympathetic listener. It seemed to come out of a past that had vanished, and conjured up a present and a future that bore no relation to our own lives.

It was now late on Sunday night and I telephoned to a friend, who was also a friend of Guy's and a member of MI6, and told him that Guy had apparently vanished into the blue and that I thought MI5 ought to be told. When he asked why, I said I thought Guy might have defected to the Soviet Union. He was, naturally enough, incredulous, but I was insistent that something should be done and he promised, somewhat reluctantly, that he would inform MI5 of what I said. The next day I received a message from him saying that he had done so and that MI5 would be getting in touch with me.

On Sunday evening, however, I also told another friend of Guy's, who had served in MI5 during the war, and still preserved close connections with it, of what I had done. He was greatly distressed, and said he would like to see me. On Monday he came down to my house in the country, and on an almost ideally beautiful English summer day, we sat beside the river and I gave him my reasons for thinking that Guy had gone to the Soviet Union; his violent anti-Americanism, his certainty that America was about to involve us all in a Third World War, most of all the fact that he may have been and perhaps still was a Soviet agent.

He pointed out, very convincingly as it seemed to me, that these were really not very good reasons for denouncing Guy to MI5. His anti-Americanism was an attitude which was shared by many liberal-minded people and if this alone were sufficient reason to drive him to the Soviet Union, Moscow at the moment would be besieged by defectors seeking asylum. On the other hand, my belief that he might be a Soviet agent rested simply on one single remark made by him years ago and apparently never repeated to anyone else; in any case, Guy's public professions of anti-Americanism were hardly what one would expect from a professional Soviet agent. Most of all he pointed out that Guy was after all one of my, as of his, oldest friends and to make the kind of allegations I apparently proposed to make about him was not, to say the least of it, the act of a friend.

He was the Cambridge liberal conscience at its very best, reasonable, sensible, and firm in the faith that personal relations are the highest of all human values. He reminded me of E. M. Forster's famous statement that if he had to choose between betraying his country or betraying his friend, he hoped he would have the courage to betray his country. I said that in the appalling political circumstances under which we lived, to betray one's country might mean betraying innumerable other friends and it might also mean betraying one's wife and one's family. I said Forster's antithesis was a false one. One's country was not some abstract conception which it might be relatively easy to sacrifice for the sake of an individual; it was itself made up of a dense network of individual and social relationships in which loyalty to one particular person formed only a single strand. In that case, he said, I was being rather irrational because after all Guy had told me he was a spy a very long time ago and I had not thought it necessary to tell anyone. I said that perhaps I was a very irrational person; but until then I had not really been convinced that Guy had been telling the truth. Now I was, and I was tired of the deceit he had practised over so many years and was only anxious to get rid of all my doubts and suspicions and speculations and pass them on to those whose business it was to say what they were worth.

He pointed out, with some force, that they were not likely to think them worth much; he even gently hinted, out of his own experience, that they might even wonder what on earth I was up to in coming to them with so curious a story. I could not help wondering if this would have been his own reaction when he was a member of MI5 himself and for a moment I had a sense of how profoundly English he was; but I repeated that I now felt that the only thing I could do was to tell the security authorities what I thought I knew as fully and precisely as I could and leave to them what use, if any, they might wish to make of it. At least it would not be my problem any more.

And so we left. He did not disguise his disapproval of what I was going to do. I spent the night in some misery and marvelled at the wonderful web of trickery and deceit Guy had woven around himself and wondered even now if I was not being foolish in believing a single word he had ever said. And yet, despite all this, and despite my conversation of that afternoon, I somehow recovered something of my conviction of the previous evening that Guy had, for whatever reason, gone to the Soviet Union, and rather irrationally this somehow cheered me up and I went to sleep.

Cheerfulness, however, did not last for long. I felt both alarmed and despondent when the next day I went up to London and made my way to MI5. I could not help reflecting on the process of events which, since my Oxford days, had finally brought me to the extraordinary position of laying information to the security authorities against one of my best friends, and on the almost total transformation in society, and perhaps in myself, this implied. It was as if somewhere along the line continuity had been broken and something new and strange had emerged, so that I hardly knew myself or the world I lived in.

At MI5 I was taken into the presence of an officer whom I had known during the war and who had also known Guy well. For a moment this made things seem easier; it was as if it was all in the family. But it also made me feel even more foolish and the whole affair more improbable; this was not the kind of thing that happened between friends. I felt as if, from afar, Guy were exercising his gift of introducing the element of farce into everything he did, however serious or even disastrous it might be.

But this sense quickly passed when, after a few questions, I began my story and I became aware of the intense seriousness with which it was listened to. I had expected surprise or even incredulity rather than this atmosphere of concentrated, even strained, attention. After all, it was a very improbable story; all I really had to say was that Guy had been absent for four days and that from this I had deduced that he had gone to Moscow.

And here this particular story really ends, for what I had to tell them at MI5 was the same story that I have told here. But when I had finished, feeling, as one always does under such circumstances, that what I had to say sounded extraordinarily thin and unconvincing, there was a long silence. Then the officer, who was the head of the department concerned, gave me a curious look; I shall never be quite certain what it meant. After a moment he said, in a detached and matter-of-fact voice:

"Of course, you knew that Guy did not go alone?"

It was certainly the last question I had expected and for a moment I was too bewildered to reply. Then I said, rather foolishly:

"You mean that Guy really has gone?"

"Yes."

"And that someone else has gone too?"

"Yes."

"Who is it?" I said.

"Donald Maclean. They went together."

Then I realized with a terrible sinking of the heart that everything I had thought about Guy was true; but that matters were even worse than I thought. They seemed even worse when I emerged from the office and in the street saw the headlines in the evening papers announcing that two British diplomats had vanished into thin air.

Five

IT might be thought that Guy's disappearing act would
have confirmed all the suspicions I had ever had about
him. In fact, it did not do so, and indeed it was surrounded by so much mystery that it merely raised a
multitude of further questions. After his initial flight
from England, and landing in France, all trace of Guy,
and of Maclean, had been lost, and despite all the investi-
gations that were set on foot, there was not the slightest
clue to their whereabouts, or to why Guy in particular
had taken so desperate a step. Maclean's case was
different. He had every reason for flight; but, except for
old friendship, there was no reason to connect Guy's case
with his, and, after the event, there were so many different
accounts of Guy's behaviour after his return from
Washington that one could quite reasonably believe that
he had acted on impulse rather than deliberate design.
Had Maclean appealed to Guy in his trouble and had Guy
merely assisted him to leave England, with the intention
of returning himself later? He had telephoned to W. H.
Auden in Ischia; had he, for reasons of his own, intended to
visit him and take a Mediterranean holiday? Was there any
reason to believe that he and Maclean were still together,
or would remain together, or that their joint disappearance
had been anything except a coincidence? Everything
seemed to point to the fact that Guy's decision to leave
had been taken on the spur of the moment; was it conceivable that, in the short time left to him, he could have
so quickly and efficiently made all the plans and arrangements required to carry them across the Channel without
leaving behind any clue to their destination?

Today, when so much more is known about their disappearance, and the part which Kim Philby played in it, and Guy himself is dead in Moscow, it is difficult to believe that one could ever have had any doubts about the answer to such questions. But at the time I was certainly not alone in doing so. The police, the security services, the press of all Europe scoured the continent in an effort to identify the whereabouts of the missing diplomats; who was I to be sure of what had happened, when so many others were not? It is not an easy thing to accept that one of one's oldest friends is a spy, even if he once told you that he was; in Guy's case I felt justified, for friendship's sake, in allowing him the benefit of every doubt so long as it was still possible to believe in his innocence, though perhaps innocence is not quite the right word. It would have been hard at any time to think of Guy as innocent. All one hoped for was that it would not be necessary to think the worst of him. I preferred to regard his disappearance as an unsolved mystery; sometimes I used to repeat to myself Browning's lines:

> *What's become of Waring*
> *Since he gave us all the slip,*
> *Chose land-travel or seafaring,*
> *Boots and chest, or staff and scrip,*
> *Rather than pace up and down*
> *Any longer London-Town?*

Indeed it was perhaps not inappropriate to apply the poem to Guy. There was a real affinity between him and the poem's original inspiration, the swashbuckling, vainglorious biographer of Byron and Shelley who entranced all his literary friends with his tales of derring-do in outlandish parts of the world and his hints of dark

213

and unspeakable mysteries in his life. Only what Trelawney related as legend, Guy turned into farce.

Guy's disappearance also had other, more direct consequences which were rather different from anything I might have expected. I had made my statement to MI5 in the belief, or the hope, that having once unburdened my conscience, I might dismiss him and his affairs from my mind. It was like Guy that by a characteristic oversight he should have made so easy an escape impossible; one might almost have thought he had done it on purpose.

His telephone call to my wife, on the morning of his disappearance, had been made from the Reform Club. It was a long and expensive call and Guy had forgotten to pay for it; but it had been easy for the club to trace, and the amount owing in Guy's name, together with the time and date of the call and my telephone number in the country, had been posted on the members' notice board at the entrance to the club. And there the notice remained until it was found by some enterprising journalist, who promptly and accurately deduced that this long personal call was the last Guy was known to have made before leaving the country. Surely it must contain some clue to the mystery of his disappearance?

The results, for me, and even more for my wife, who had actually received the call, were disastrous. My identity, my address in the country, and my telephone number were soon known to the Press of the entire country, whose representatives descended upon my house at Sonning as if some notorious criminal, or his accomplices, were in hiding there. Their cars packed my drive; the doorbell and telephone rang incessantly; they took photographs of my wife, myself, and my children from every conceivable angle. They camped in the village and besieged the local pubs and pursued their enquiries in all the village shops; they pressed chocolates and half crowns on my children in their search for information about Guy, and my children were only too happy to exercise their imagination on satisfying their curiosity. My wife's slightly incoherent account of her even more incoherent conversation with Guy only convinced the Press that there was something to conceal; indeed, even we had to admit that it didn't sound very convincing. Photographed as *Mother of Four Knew Burgess*, she became a regular feature of the daily papers, which somehow succeeded in importing an indefinable air of kinkiness into the relationship. Some members of the Press simply took this for granted; one who by some means penetrated into the house introduced himself with the words: "It's all right to talk to me, Mrs Rees. I'm bi-sexual myself."

This form of persecution lasted for several weeks. It seemed as if pandemonium had suddenly descended on our lives, and we learned to live with journalists as one does with bugs in the walls; it was impossible to drive them out. For the Cold War was raging; the "Case of the Missing Diplomats" had become a world-wide sensation, threatening our national security, and we found ourselves at the centre of it. Each day new stories appeared in the Press, and each day, like modern Scarlet Pimpernels, Guy and Maclean, together or apart, were reported to have been seen in different parts of Europe. They had been seen in Paris, they had been seen in Monte Carlo, they had been seen in Berlin, they had been seen in Prague; once, to my dismay, I was rung up in the middle of the night to be told that Guy had been seen leaving Reading station, presumably on his way to visit me at Sonning. Amid considerable publicity, and at great expense, the *Daily Express* hired the redoubtable Colonel Pinto, "the greatest spy hunter in the world", to conduct a search for the missing pair that would take him throughout the length and breadth of Europe without discovering a trace of them. Each item of news, or what purported to be news, provoked a fresh barrage of telephone calls or visits by reporters to ask what one thought about it; for the most remarkable feature of the case was that there was really no news at all, and any kind of comment, or even a refusal to comment, was eagerly seized on as a means of stimulating and appeasing public curiosity.

It was clear that I was not going to be allowed to forget Guy very easily, however much I might wish to; he had become a kind of permanent shadow who never left my side. Sometimes I even had hallucinations in which I suddenly glimpsed his tall, slightly hunched figure, disappearing round the corner of the street. Even when, after some months, the appetite for news of press and public began to die of starvation, some stray item of gossip or rumour would revive it, and once again the telephone would ring, reporters would present themselves at the door, and the great machine of publicity lumber into action. For the truth was that the case of the missing diplomats had all the elements of one of those stories of crime and detection in which public interest never really dies, and it had an uncanny capacity for keeping itself alive. It had treachery and deceit, it had politics, it had espionage, it had sex, of an off-beat kind, it had the flavour of high society which people mistakenly associate with diplomatic circles, and it had, almost to excess, those touches of the eccentric and bizarre which have been compulsory in all detective stories since Sherlock Holmes first made them possible. What writer could create a hero, or a villain, whose favourite food was, like Guy's, a dried fish which, in the heart of London, he hung out of his window on a piece of string and occasionally hauled in, in order to cut himself a slice and satisfy his hunger?

Most of all, perhaps, it had as its heart and centre a profound psychological puzzle, which was how it could be that two young Englishmen, both of them gifted and intelligent, and of the most irreproachable social background and upbringing, should suddenly, for whatever motive, abandon everything to which their privileged position entitled them and take off into the blue. One would be hard enough to explain, but *two* of them? It made of the case not only a puzzle which, until the truth was known, provided an almost unlimited field for speculation, but, vaguely, a kind of threat; it made people feel that in a society in which such things were possible, anything was possible, and there was nothing one could be sure of, as if everywhere unseen abysses yawned beneath one's feet. The missing diplomats (how strange it was to think of Guy in the image of a diplomat!) not only evoked the kind of curiosity which makes one want to know the end of a detective story; it made people uneasy until they knew the answer.

For the time being, however, there was no answer to be had, and the story remained a mystery. But it was not only a mystery in itself, it suggested other possible mysteries. For if one assumed that Guy and Maclean had been enemy agents, was it likely or possible that they had worked in total isolation, without collaborators or accomplices; if there had been two of them, would there not also have been more? As months went by, it became evident that at least one possible accomplice existed in the person of the mysterious Third Man, who was believed to have given warning that Maclean was to be taken in for interrogation and so had provoked his, and Guy's, flight; but it had been authoritatively announced in Parliament that this hypothetical figure was not Kim Philby, Guy's friend and late host in Washington, who had indeed come under suspicion but after a rigorous enquiry by the security service had been totally exonerated.

What else could one do but accept such a verdict, delivered on such impeccable authority? Yet the whole of my association with Guy, together with the fact of his flight, had by now left me with an incurable disposition to doubt and suspect all impeccable authorities. If I had, for so many years, dismissed his own assertion that he was, or had been a spy, it was precisely because so many of Guy's friends and intimates had been in a position to verify his credentials and had presumably found no reason to doubt them; if their judgement was not to be trusted, whose could be? Who was I, who had so much less information at my command, to think that mine was any better? To do so seemed both presumptuous and to conjure up such a miasma of doubt and suspicion that one could put one's trust in no one.

Such mysteries, I decided, were not for me to solve; it would be impossible to live at all if one felt that at the very heart of the country's security system there lay some fatal flaw which constantly exposed it to error and disaster. It would be as if some explorer, having accidentally stumbled on some country's most secret shrine, had discovered that its altar was made of papier maché and its priests were a gang of devil worshippers—or perhaps merely grinning imbeciles. The whole thing was too absurd.

So at least I argued to myself; and in any case why should I worry if the altar was hollow, so long as I did not worship at it myself? Espionage and counter espionage were at best some kind of absurd game to which no rational person could attach any serious significance. Yet in fact, at some irrational level, all the circumstances of Guy's disappearance had left me with a sense that somewhere something was appallingly wrong and that if only I tried hard enough and thought deeply enough I should be able to find the clue to what it was.

In part this was an effect of the reception I had been given by MI5. When I first told them that I believed Guy had gone to Moscow, it was largely out of a sense of desperation and urgency. Guy had hardly been two days gone, and I had felt that it was still not too late to prevent a calamity, even that, if only the means and resources were available, I myself could follow his trail and might possibly prevail on him to return. At least, I felt that if anyone could do so I could, if the opportunity were made available.

Perhaps this was too much to expect; responsible organizations do not take action on the intuitions of some uninformed outsider or respond to a slightly hysterical message out of the blue. What puzzled me then, and continued to puzzle me later was that, as far as Guy was concerned, my message must have been the first intimation they received that, as far as he was concerned, anything was amiss; could it really be that I alone, among all those who had known him, and some even better than I, was the only one who had ever had suspicions of him or any knowledge that threw doubt on his reliability? It seemed to me impossible that this could be so, and of course in fact it was not so; only unfortunately those who, like Kim Philby, had shared that knowledge were precisely those who had most interest in concealing it.

There was a further aspect of MI5's behaviour which made me feel uneasy. I had always felt that if at any time prior to Guy's disappearance I had told MI5 what I thought I knew about Guy, my story would have been received with polite scepticism, even incredulity, as the product of an overheated imagination stimulated by reading too much about Soviet espionage. But now that I had done so, and at the very moment of Guy's disappearance, it must surely have seemed to them something more than a coincidence; why, after so many years of silence, should a person like myself, with no professional interest in the case, suddenly volunteer information which certainly did no credit to one of my best friends and not very much to myself? The questions they put to me at my interview, indeed their very manner of asking them, made an oddly ambivalent impression; I seemed to detect in them a note of—what was it?—of something very nearly approaching moral disapproval, as if I had acted in a manner unbecoming a gentleman, combined with a hardly concealed disbelief in my motives for offering information at precisely the moment when it was too late. It would have been too much to say that they treated me as if I myself were an object of suspicion; it was simply that they conveyed the impression that, from their point of view, there was something very peculiar about the whole performance.

I had been taken aback by their manner; somehow it was not what I had expected. It was almost as if they resented my intervention and I were an added embarrassment in a situation which was already embarrassing enough. On the other hand, it hardly seemed to matter what they thought of me. I had told them all I knew, and what use, if any, they made of the information was no concern of mine. And yet, just as they seemed suspicious of me, so I in turn was not without suspicion of them. I felt as if I had intruded into some complicated game they were playing and had made some unorthodox move which interfered with its smooth progress; their reaction,

I felt, was to remove the intruder as painlessly as possible and reduce the effect of his intervention to a minimum.

Beneath all this was another consideration which made me feel vaguely uneasy. It had become clear that Maclean, at least, had certainly been engaged in espionage; and whatever doubts one might have had about what part Guy had played in his operations, there was no doubt that he had been willing to assist Maclean to escape the consequences of being found out. I myself felt sure that their behaviour had its origins in the days when many years ago they had been communists together in Cambridge; the most natural assumption to make was that at that time they had both been recruited into the Soviet espionage system.

All this seemed plain; but if this were so, then it also seemed highly unlikely that Guy and Maclean were the only ones among their contemporaries at Cambridge to have been recruited. The Hiss case had shown that in America in the 30s large numbers of young intellectuals had been enlisted into the Soviet espionage system; they had been, *mutatis mutandis*, of the same class and social background as Guy and Maclean, and they had had considerable success in penetrating the United States government; in this sense at least there was a basis of fact to the extravagances and demagoguery of Senator McCarthy's wild accusations. Was it likely that in Britain the Soviet Union would have been satisfied with some lesser objective and have been content with the recruitment of two young men of whom, at the moment, it would have been impossible to say whether they would have been of any future use? It seemed highly probable that if Guy and Maclean had been recruited as spies, so had others, and that, if they had vanished, others remained.

But who? I had the uneasy feeling that the likeliest place to look was in the ranks of the security services themselves.

There seemed to be only one other conclusion to draw. If one assumed that Maclean's value had been in the high-level political information to which he had access, then Guy's would have consisted in the extremely varied and comprehensive knowledge he had acquired, largely as a result of personal relationships, of the British security services. Of the two types of information, I had no doubt which would have been considered of most value by the Soviet espionage system; nor which was likely to have the most practical, and the most deplorable results.

Political or diplomatic information, however secret, is very rarely of great value; certainly of no greater value than the information available to any enterprising, pertinacious and intelligent journalist. Moreover, it is very rarely reliable, in the sense that it can be acted upon, because it is concerned with questions of policy, and policy is always subject to change and also to conflicting interpretations. In the great game of espionage, the information which is most highly valued is that which enables one to identify the players on the opposite side; that is to say, the members of the enemy espionage system. In the same way, the highest degree of secrecy attaches to the identity of the members of one's own team. That is why espionage is for the most part a self-defeating activity, in which the two opposing sides fight a fierce fratricidal battle behind closed doors with the ultimate objective of wiping the other side out. Any information which confers an advantage in the battle is of the very highest value; moreover, since it refers to individual human beings, it has the technical advantage of being concrete, detailed, and subject to verification; it can even be subjected to experiment. Moreover, it can be acted upon in the most direct and practical manner; that is to say, it can be used to destroy the reputation, credit, honour, and in critical cases even the lives of one's opponents. I had no doubt that Guy was admirably equipped to supply this particular kind of information; and also that it was information which could have the most disastrous results for the individuals whom it concerned.

But it was also true that his main source of such information was the friends and acquaintances he cultivated so assiduously in the British intelligence services; and that among them were several who had been contemporaries of his at Cambridge, that is to say, that they belonged to precisely those intellectual and radical circles to which Guy and Maclean had themselves. Given that Guy was a spy, the question for any alert intelligence officer to ask at this point was whether his sources of information were conscious or unconscious; whether they had merely been indiscreet or insecure in their conversations with him, or whether they, or some of them, had collaborated with him in the common task of penetrating the British intelligence services.

Why did I feel that our security services were incapable of seriously addressing such a question to themselves? I should have found it very difficult to give any very rational or convincing explanation, even to myself. It was simply the sense that the members of our intelligence services were, in so many cases, so closely bound together by ties of origin, upbringing, education and class that they were effectively inhibited from facing the possibility that there were traitors in their midst. Of course, in the case of Maclean, and possibly of Guy, it had already been shown that there were persons of their own kind who were capable of such treachery; but this in itself was so unnatural and monstrous that it could only constitute a unique case, never again to be repeated.

Our security services, in fact, seemed to me a microcosm of that "great capitalist class", now in the process of intellectual disintegration, whose structure and organization, modes of behaviour and thought, I had found so alien when I first went to Oxford. In those days I had devoted much time and thought to studying them; they had fascinated me as the discovery of some hitherto unknown animal species might fascinate a zoologist. I had wondered at how easily they accepted the assumption that they were destined to form as it were "the committee of management" of the country of which they were the most privileged citizens, believing indeed that their very privileges, not merely of wealth or birth, but of intellect and ability, gave them the right to be so. And in a sense they had been right; but even then, now nearly a quarter of a century ago, I had felt that there was a kind of worm at the heart of the glossy apple, ruddy and rounded to perfection, which they held out to one for one's admiration. The worm, I had thought, had been the inordinate and predominant importance which they had ascribed to personal relationships, organized into a philosophical and ethical system, and even into a system of government. In *Principia Ethica* G. E. Moore had appeared to give an absolute value to such an attitude; but Moore had been misunderstood, and even Moore, it seemed to me, had never done more than erect his personal intuitions into a philosophy. However deeply we may feel the value of personal relationships it is impossible to abstract and divorce them from other, impersonal factors in our lives, both material and spiritual, which are of equal or of even greater importance, and indeed if we do so we may deprive personal relations themselves of the roots which give them their real life and vitality.

The exaggerated, indeed, supreme importance ascribed to personal relationships in Cambridge, as at Oxford, at the end of the 1920s, could be interpreted as the mark of a society which was becoming increasingly incapable of mastering, whether in theory or practice, the problems of the real world, and in this sense it reflected the decline of a great intellectual tradition, of which G. E. Moore himself was one of the inheritors. The decline may have been due in large part to the terrible blood-letting which the British governing class had suffered in the First World War; a sharp awareness of this decline played a major part in the complex of reasons which drove Guy and many of his contemporaries into the arms of communism. They were inspired, not so much by sympathy with the sufferings of the working class at a time of capitalist crisis, as by an awareness that their own class, "the great capitalist class", could no longer find a remedy for them. Of the working class in fact they knew nothing and they worshipped it as an idol whose virtue and power they accepted on the evidence of things unseen. It was the defects and inadequacies of their own class which effected their conversion; in the Soviet Union and communism they saw a new world which they called in to restore the balance of the old.

No doubt their commitment to communism led some of them into ways which were infinitely more evil and destructive than those they had abandoned; but perhaps they were not mistaken in their perception of the declining vitality and intellectual power of the class to which they themselves belonged, even though their own conversion to communism might be only another manifestation of it. But at least they had achieved one particular insight which put them, as it were, one step ahead of those among their contemporaries who, while Guy and Maclean had become spies, had drifted, without particular conviction, into becoming counter spies. These recruits to the British intelligence service, of whom Guy used sometimes to say that they had the characteristic vices and weaknesses of "the failed intellectual", seemed to me to be fatally inhibited from solving the problems offered by Guy's and Maclean's defection by the intellectual and emotional assumptions of the class to which they belonged, and against which Guy and Maclean had revolted; by mistaken loyalties based on old friendships and intimacies, by failure to understand the inadequacy of their own attitudes and beliefs, by inability to accept that the motives which had operated in Guy's and Maclean's case might also operate in others. Perhaps indeed they might prefer that the problems might remain unsolved; for certainly the answer would reveal much about themselves as well as Guy and Maclean.

So I continued to feel that the task of unravelling the mystery of the missing diplomats was in ineffective hands; indeed, that some of those hands may have been engaged in the same kind of enterprises as Guy. I remained convinced that Guy and Maclean had not been alone in their activities, but that, for reasons which were deeply rooted in the English social system, it was unlikely that their collaborators would be discovered.

II

At the Christmas following his disappearance, I received a card, with an English postmark, from Guy. It merely sent his greetings and expressed the hope that some time we should meet again. It was at least evidence that he was still alive, though not of much else, but somehow the message did not affect me very deeply. Guy's flight had been the culmination of so many years of doubt and speculation, and had caused so much distress not only to my family and myself, but to a wide circle of his friends, that I no longer wished to see or hear any more of him. He had vanished out of my life, and when I thought of him it was rather as one thinks of a character in a novel or a play, who for some time has had the power to stir one's emotions and absorb one's interest but has no connection with the actual task of daily living.

Yet, perhaps, he still had the power of indirectly affecting my own behaviour. His disappearance, and the events which had led up to it, had somehow intensified my doubts and misgivings about the society in which I was now, it appeared, so firmly rooted. Perhaps this was because Guy, with all his eccentricities and deviations, had always seemed to me one of the most English of characters; indeed, one could not have conceived of him as being anything else than English. No doubt he was an exception, but he was also representative, an exception which proved the rule perhaps, only I could not quite make out what the rule was; unless it was that he was a part, and a significant part, of a society which, at this stage in its long history, had lost its way, and with it, the qualities which had once made it great. Perhaps his flight had only been the precursor of other flights, in different directions, which others would soon take in order to evade the realities of the world in which they were doomed to live.

There was a time, during the war, when England had seemed to recover the virtues of its past greatness. As a gunner in the ranks I had for the first time come into close, even bodily contact, which that great English working class which had so often been the object of

Marxist theory and speculation; it had touched me to see in these dockers, labourers, clerks, drunkards, gamblers, from the East End of London the same qualities of the English as we know them in the works of Shakespeare, or Fielding, or Defoe, or Dickens; the same tolerance and forbearance, the same gifts of humour and imagination, combined with the residue of something which was almost barbarism yet gave them a kind of primitive power of endurance. Yet the war itself had proved to be one more stage in a long decline, and in post-war England there was little or no evidence that the decline could be averted or halted. There were of course objective reasons, historical, political and economic, why this should be so; but history is made by men and it seemed to me that the men who effectively ruled, governed and administered England after the war were not the men required to reverse its long decline into mediocrity.

> *Be you the men your fathers were*
> *And God will save the Queen.*

They were not the men their fathers were. They were in many ways more enlightened, more humane, more civilized, more progressive, but some mysterious inner core of adjustment to the world as it really is, and not as it seems or one wishes it to be had been lost. It struck me, with an almost personal sense of involvement, that, grown to maturity, they were the men whom I had known some twenty years ago as undergraduates, and that having achieved the power and responsibility they had always assumed the right to expect, they were now unable to make effective use of them.

Perhaps Guy cast his shadow over such ideas. It had been one of his favourite themes to contrast the greatness of the Victorians, in politics, in industry, in literature, with the littleness of their descendants, and he would elaborate his theme by describing the fall of the British steel industry or the Royal Navy from their position of pre-eminence in the world, or by comparing George Eliot with E. M. Forster, or Dickens with D. H. Lawrence; nothing exemplified it better, to his mind, than the difference in sheer intellectual power between those eminent Victorians, Manning, Arnold, Newman, and their biographer, Lytton Strachey, who had chosen them as the victims of his wit and malice. It was a case, he thought, of a pigmy sneering at giants; and in that "secret" society of the Apostles at Cambridge, of which he was a member, he saw the same decline from the greatness of the English past.

Perhaps such thoughts helped to intensify in me an uneasy sense of dissatisfaction with my own life, though on the surface at least there seemed to be little reason for it. My marriage, and my children, had brought me great happiness. I had ceased to be a journalist and had joined an old friend, Henry Yorke, as a director of his family engineering business. It was a change which I found eminently satisfactory, because after the war journalism had become less and less attractive to me, while engineering introduced me to an entirely new and unfamiliar world which I found unexpectedly fascinating. My duties, which were far from arduous, were enlivened by day-to-day and almost minute-to-minute contact with Henry himself, who both as a writer and a person had something which was very near to genius, if genius means a completely individual view of life which reveals reality in an entirely new and unexpected light. To live side by side with him in the office was to see the world through a new and entirely different pair of eyes; in the course of the day he turned from Henry Yorke the businessman, much concerned with money and profit, to Henry Green the novelist, writing books between the intervals of negotiating contracts for brewing machinery and chemical plant, and he allowed me the same liberty in the use I made of my time.

In addition, as Estates Bursar of All Souls, I had been brought back into closer contact with the college, and with Oxford, than I had been for many years, though both had greatly changed from what they once were. Gone were the aesthetes and the hearties, and gone also the radicals and revolutionaries who had succeeded them; the immediate post-war generation of undergraduates was intensely serious and hardworking, far more responsible and mature than those of my own day and with no time for their kind of follies and eccentricities. Their studies came first, all the more so because the war had made England poor and economic pressures made the problem of a career very important to them. The dons also had changed; a much higher proportion were married, and the pleasures and cares of domestic life now occupied the place which had once been reserved for their pupils. The home, not the college, was now the centre of their lives, and that community in which both dons and undergraduates had played an equal part, of which not a trace remains today, was already beginning to break down.

But life at All Souls was agreeable and interesting to me at that time because of the presence of a group of young philosophers to whom their subject was a matter of consuming interest; they pursued it with a passion which other men might have devoted to girls or horses. This was odd, because their particular kind of philosophy was arid and scholastic to the last degree and was almost exclusively concerned with linguistic and semantic problems. They argued about words, and more particularly those words of which, because they are a matter of common usage, everyone thinks he understands the meaning, with the same intensity as Browning's grammarian settled Hoti's business. Under the influence of a remarkable man, J. L. Austin, himself once a Fellow of All Souls, who by moral rather than intellectual power ruled them as a stern schoolmaster rules unruly pupils, they pursued this philosophical game with almost religious devotion, and nothing could have been more curious than the fervour and piety with which they joined in his profound enquiries into the exact meaning, in a multitude of different contexts, of such words as "is", "if" and "not".

Their intellectual labours may have been arid but they themselves were not; on the contrary, they had the gaiety and lightheartedness of the single-minded. They were like young men who were engaged in a crusade, who felt that at last the mysteries of the universe were to be, if not solved, at least eliminated as the product of mere verbal confusions, and they applied themselves to this process of mental hygiene with the zeal of a highly efficient municipal cleansing department. Error, not truth, was their quarry, and they hunted it down relentlessly in every word or phrase one spoke; but like Austin himself, they brought to the chase a certain dry humour and wit which made it as much of a pastime as an intellectual exercise.

There was an absurdity about their entire enterprise, and their devotion to it, which gave it a certain eccentric charm, and to me at least made their company highly entertaining and stimulating. Their conversation enlivened my visits to the college to attend to its financial affairs, which was largely a matter of trying to reconcile our excessive income with an inadequate expenditure. For largely through the efforts of my predecessor, Geoffrey Faber, the college was rich. He had nursed its estates through the agricultural depression of the 20s and 30s, had undertaken large schemes of capital investment, built housing estates and roads, so that when I succeeded him they were in an extremely prosperous condition. There had been a time when no rent could be low enough to attract a tenant to some of the college's estates, and the college had to resort to direct farming; Whitsundoles, a farm in Romney Marsh, was a name that resounded mournfully at every college meeting because of the losses which had been incurred on it.

By 1952, when I succeeded Faber, the college estates had increased enormously in value, both because of the general prosperity of English agriculture and because of Faber's wise policies. One of the first problems which met me as Estates Bursar was how best to dispose of a sum of over £1,000,000, which had been received in compensation for the public acquisition of its lands in Edgeware, a part of the college's original endowment by its founder, Archbishop Chichele. But colleges like All Souls, which have enjoyed a continuous existence since the Middle Ages, have a long communal memory which often proves stronger than the rational intentions of the living. They remember the bad times as well as the good, and tend to regard any increase in prosperity as purely fortuitous and accidental. When it was proposed that the college should seek a further increase in its wealth by investing its funds in equities, there was a sense that, for five hundred years, only the land had kept the college alive through all its varying fortunes. I could not help being impressed, as if by the voice of some ancient wisdom, by a remark of Lord Brand's, chairman of Lazard's and a director of the Bank of England, who was one of the college's shrewdest financial advisors: "If there had been such a thing as equities in the Middle Ages," he said scornfully, "there wouldn't be a college in existence in Oxford today." How astonishing it was, in the middle of the twentieth century, to hear one who was a master of all the mysteries of contemporary high finance, speak as if, so far as Oxford was concerned, what had been valid in the Middle Ages was still valid today! It was an assertion that, for a college, survival and continuity are more important than profit and that its primary duty is, like the land, to live for ever.

The land! When I first became Estates Bursar, it still constituted the main source of the college's wealth. In those days, the college estates consisted of some thirty thousand acres which extended as far as Yorkshire in the north, Kent in the south, Norfolk in the east and Shropshire in the west. I found the supervision of the estates, under the guidance and tuition of the college's extremely efficient agents, an absorbing and fascinating occupation. Like Henry Yorke's engineering business, it brought me into contact with an aspect of England I had not known before; in this case the land, not as an object of beauty, or pleasure, or art, but as a means, and the most ancient means of all, by which men make their living. Sometimes, talking to the tenant of some bleak hill farm in Yorkshire, the wind from the moors whistling round my ears as I listened to his complaints, to his requests for a new milking parlour or some improvement to his house, I used to remember my grandfather's little farm in Wales and think it was certainly better to be the tenant of a wealthy Oxford college than to depend on the spendthrift eccentricities of the Pryses of Plas Gogerddan. I could hardly believe that on the fat pastures of Romney Marsh an acre could carry eight of its ponderous Kentish sheep while one of our tender Welsh ones could hardly survive on eight acres of Plynlimon's sparse mountain grass. I used to recite to myself *The War Song of Dinas Fawr:*

> *The Mountain sheep are sweeter*
> *But the valley sheep are fatter,*
> *We therefore deemed it meeter*
> *To carry off the latter.*

My wife and children; a pleasant house with a large garden on the Thames; a business that was in itself interesting and allowed me leisure to write what I wished; the academic life of All Souls, combined with the mundane realities of managing the college properties; all this was enough to provide me with an active and satisfactory life and should, I suppose, have been sufficient to keep me happy. And yet it was not. Somehow my life had taken a path I had not intended and chance had cast me in a part which I could not play with conviction. I seemed to have become a different person and I regretted the one I had been. I was not unhappy but I was vaguely dissatisfied and disorientated, as if forces beyond my control had set me on a course which I had not chosen for myself and from which henceforth there would be no deviation.

Such feelings, I am sure, were quite unjustified. In my case at least, the difficulties of living had never arisen out of pursuing too settled and regular a course, but rather out of failure to remain on any course at all except for the briefest periods. It was always the unexpected and not the expected that had happened; even my marriage had taken me by surprise; and winds, storms or soft and scented breezes had never come from the quarter in which one had looked for them. There was no reason for me to regret that, for the time being, life had treated me almost too kindly or to have felt that I was overburdened with security. All I had to do was to wait for the hand of chance to reveal itself once again, and in the meantime enjoy the good things which life had given me.

And indeed in a way chance did show its hand and in a way which could not have been more surprising; only this time it required my own collaboration to produce its effect, and this was disastrous. There is a particular class of people, to which I belong, which if offered a choice between two particular courses of action will almost invariably choose what is from their own point of view the wrong one, because they do not understand what they themselves are like and therefore miscalculate the most important factor in the situation.

On this occasion chance showed its hand in the form of a letter from Aberystwyth asking me if I were willing to be considered for the appointment of Principal of the University College of Wales. If I had been wise, I would have recognized in the letter a most dangerous form of seduction; and if I had had any sense I would have realized that such letters, particularly if they come from Wales, are never quite what they seem and are usually the product of long hours of not entirely disinterested thought and deliberation. I should have been warned, and I should have been even more on my guard if I had known that, though the letter did not come directly from him, its writing concealed the fine Welsh hand of Dr Thomas Jones, once Under-Secretary to the Cabinet, adviser to two Prime Ministers, now President of the University College and a kind of *éminence grise* in the management of the affairs of the Welsh people; for Dr Jones was a skilled manipulator of men and situations and nothing he did was ever as simple as it might seem.

I did not, however, try to decipher the implications of the letter, because, on first reading, it simply appeared absurd. Why should anyone think that, after so many years of absence, I should return to that bleak little town in which I had been born and that now seemed as remote as the childhood I had spent there? It was like being asked to return to the nursery and play again with the toys which had been discarded since infancy, and all the more so since after leaving Wales I had thought of it as the land of a dying language and culture which could no longer satisfy anyone except the very young and the very old.

Yet the letter obscurely appealed to some confused instinct within me which told me that precisely now, after so many years, was perhaps the time when I should return. I was even inclined to flatter myself that perhaps my very absence might have given me something to offer, in the way of experience or knowledge which I should not have had if I had not lived away from Wales for so long. Had not Dr Jones himself entitled a book of his *The Native Never Returns*, because the native who does return is a different person from the one who left? Might it not be that he and the native who had never left his home might together achieve something different and better than either could have done in isolation? There was something stimulating, even exciting in the idea that there, in Aberystwyth, stood an institute of learning which had already played a large part in the life of the Welsh people and which now one might, with patience and persistence, help to play an even greater part. I was sufficiently persuaded of the value of university education, and especially the education of young Welshmen, to believe that this was something worth doing, and I thought that perhaps a university which genuinely fulfilled its function was perhaps of all things the one which my people most needed.

Such indeed had been the hope of the original founders of the university college, the first of its kind in Wales,

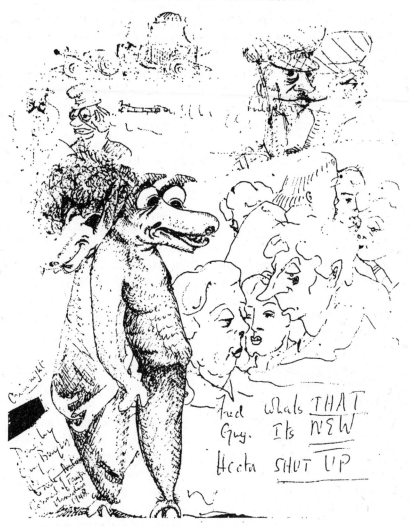

CRISIS NIGHT

Drawing by Guy Burgess, done at the Council of Foreign
Ministers, Paris, 1948.

at the end of the nineteenth century. It had been founded by private subscription and on the pennies of the poor, and had been intended to give the Welsh people educational and intellectual opportunities which had hitherto been denied them, to show them wider horizons than the confines of the farm or the coal-pit, and to enable them to play a larger part in the life of the world than had been open to them until then. Its founders had been inspired by a generous spirit; they had believed passionately in the native intelligence of the Welsh people and their capacity to achieve a wider and more self-critical culture than that of the mine, the chapel and the farm. They had dreamed of breeding a new race of Welshmen who, through the cultivation of the mind, might raise themselves and their people out of the slough of ignorance and poverty in which they had languished for centuries and out of which they had only recently begun to struggle. They had even hoped that the university might bring to Wales something of that sweetness and light which Matthew Arnold had believed was the quality which differentiated culture from barbarism.

It had been a noble dream, translated into reality in the face of immense difficulties and obstacles. If it had been only incompletely realized that only meant that there was still work to be done, and why should I not help to do it? Most of all, perhaps, I was tempted by the thought that it might depend very much on myself whether it was done; for after so many years in which, as it seemed to me, I had been a mere onlooker on life, never wholly committed to or engaged in any occupation I had adopted, was it not perhaps time that I should put my hand to something for which I myself would be responsible? I had been don, journalist, a traveller about Europe, soldier, business man, bursar, and in each of these occupations it had seemed to me that I was only acting a part. I could have said with Rimbaud: *Je suis un autre.* Was it not time to commit myself?

It was the temptation of action, on however modest a scale. But there were also other temptations. There was the feeling that in Wales, amid its hills and streams, my children might enjoy the same kind of childhood as I had myself enjoyed, as if a lost paradise awaited them there, like the lost counties engulfed under the waters of Cardigan Bay, which only children could recover; I had never quite lost the belief that, whatever might be the case for grown men, Wales was the only country for children.

When I talked to my wife of such ideas, she was astounded and looked at me with that incredulous look, so familiar to me, which meant that she thought I had once again taken leave of my senses. For her, there could be no possible attraction in a voluntary migration to a small Welsh town, hardly more than a village, whose chief architectural features were a decrepit pier, twenty-two Nonconformist chapels, and the vast Victorian Gothic hotel, a monument to the nineteenth century railway boom, in which the University College of Wales had found its first home. Moreover, and partly because of me, she thought of the Welsh as of some primitive tribe which spoke an unintelligible language, practised savage rites and customs, and was in general shiftless, untrustworthy and hostile to strangers. To her, Aberystwyth represented a kind of Welsh ghetto, in which she would feel as much at home as in some Patagonian settlement full of naked savages.

When I showed her the letter, her first reaction was, like mine, that the proposal was of course totally absurd and not worth a second's thought. But women have more

239

generous instincts than men and when, to her astonishment, she realized that the prospect of returning to
Wales, for reasons she did not understand and certainly
did not agree with, genuinely attracted me, she said,
rather doubtfully, that of course if I knew what I wanted
I must do as I wished. She acted out of the kind of
generosity which in the end hurts oneself as well as
others, and by self-sacrifice made it possible for me to
persist in my folly.

I replied to the letter that I was willing to be considered
for the appointment, though not if the college had any
other candidate in view. In due course, after an interview
with the college council in which I suddenly felt that
perhaps my wife's view of my countrymen had a certain
justification, I found myself charged with the duties of
Principal of the University College of Wales.

III

Accordingly, in the summer of 1952, we went into
residence at Aberystwyth, in a charming little Welsh
Plas, or manor house, which stood on a hill which
commanded a magnificent view of the entire sweep of
Cardigan Bay down to the last glimpse of St. David's Head
in the south. I had known the house as a child, when I
had been taken there by my mother and it was still the
property of a typically feckless family of Welsh squires.
As is the normal fate of their class, they had fallen on evil
days, and the *Plas* had only recently been acquired by
the college, as a residence for its principal.

The house should have been, as it used to be, delightful,
but it was not, and in this respect it seemed to typify the
dead hand which a nascent Welsh Establishment had
laid upon its own country and its own people. Its little
park, that extended down the grassy slope of the hill on

which it stood, was screened by a wide curtain of woods
through which a mountain stream descended in a series of
miniscule cascades. Buzzards hovered and swooped over-
head; the woods were alive with red squirrels and in the
mild climate of the Welsh coast the roses bloomed until
Christmas.

But something had gone wrong. The modest grey stone
of the house, that had once stood on the hill like an
outcrop of the rock on which it was built, had been clad
in a cement of so dazzling, so synthetic, a white that it
seemed an affront to the green and grey of the landscape
and of the sea that lapped the shore below. The sloping
lawn outside the house had been geometrically dissected
into botanical family beds, which gave it the appearance
of a municipal park, and within, all the house's modest
architectural features, its picture rails, pediments, cor-
nices, wainscots had been ruthlessly stripped away in the
process of renovation, so that each room presented the
same blank repetitive surface to the eye. It was as if some
mad geometrician had been at work, who had insisted
that nothing should remain which would mar the math-
ematical perfection of straight lines and rectangles, and
the result had been to achieve, in this old house where
centuries had once left their mark, an almost Euclidean
austerity which nothing could soften or domesticate. It
made my wife cry; while I was slightly disconcerted to
find that this ruthless work of reconstruction had been
carried out regardless both of expense and of the strict
building controls which were then in force; licences, it
seemed, were a matter which did not affect the Principal.

This fine disregard for legality is something which
comes very easily to the Welsh who, having endured an
alien rule for so long, regard its laws as something which
it is a duty to circumvent rather than obey. In the case of

the Principal, especially, who in so small a community as Aberystwyth enjoyed an almost feudal pre-eminence, it was taken for granted that he was not subject to the petty restrictions imposed by an alien bureaucracy in Whitehall. I found such an attitude embarrassing; to my wife, with her English respect for the law, it seemed positively immoral, and all the more so because it was thought natural that she should benefit by it most of all. She spent much time and effort in trying to persuade tradespeople—coal merchants, butchers, grocers—that rationing applied to her just as much as anyone else. She did not have much success; they simply refused to believe that she meant what she said and she continued to be the unwilling beneficiary of a black market which worked in strict accordance with one's position in the social system.

My wife was all the more disconcerted, indeed positively alarmed, by such procedures because they were combined with an intense curiosity about our domestic and private lives. It was a genuine shock to her to discover that an elderly emeritus professor, and member of the college Council, should make enquiries of our coal merchant about the size of our coal bill; I tried to explain that in a tribe, where the affairs of one are the affairs of all, there is no such thing as a private life, but she was apt to reply that this was all very well if one happened to be one of the tribe but it was not easy to bear if one were not. She had the native English sense that men and women are individuals who, within the limits of the law, should be allowed to pursue their own interests without interference by anyone else; she found herself among people for whom totem and taboo were superior not only to the law but to the individual.

There was material for high comedy in such a situation; my wife found herself in the position of a Daisy Miller, a visitor from the New World, whose innocence cannot adapt itself to the unspoken assumptions and complicated rituals of an ancient folk culture. But the comedy was hard to appreciate because at its heart lay the hardly veiled hostility with which her new neighbours regarded the alien stranger who had come among them; an attitude expressed at its crudest and most direct by the local drunkard and ne'er-do-well who, lounging against the railings of the town clock in the mean little square at the top of the High Street, never failed to murmur *English Bitch!* beneath his breath whenever my wife should happen to pass. This was indeed extravagant enough to be comic; she found it more offensive when the more genteel and better-bred local ladies ostentatiously spoke Welsh whenever she was present, even though normally they would have spoken in English.

It was perhaps inevitable that, quite apart from racial and social differences, such antagonisms should arise, for she was everything that those around her were not. She was young and pretty and filled with gaiety and energy; love, laughter and work were what came most naturally to her. Aberystwyth was a town of the middle aged and the old and its ladies were absorbed in the monotonous and repetitive social life of the town and the college, in which the pettiness of provincial life was combined with the acrimony of academic dissension. Gossip, morning coffee, tea parties at which dainty sandwiches and sugared cakes were handed round on lace doilies, academic and religious functions which were both equally impregnated with a Nonconformist gloom as thick as the sea fog which sometimes filled the streets of the town, were the only social diversions offered her. In such a society she was so much a fish out of water, a bird in a Methodist cage, that no basis for mutual understanding existed. She found her only natural allies among the students, who like her were young and eager for life and oppressed by the obsolescent orthodoxies of their elders, and to their affairs she devoted herself with an admirable energy which only earned her further disapproval.

For in the social and academic hierarchy of Aberystwyth students occupied the lowest position. They were regarded as youthful and not strictly human barbarians, hobbledehoys from the mining valleys and the farms, whose only function was to accept with gratitude the instruction handed down to them from above. Little or no provision was made by the college for any form of social activity, except athletic, outside their studies. Their union consisted of cramped and dilapidated premises that would not have accommodated a tenth of their number and resembled a rather sleazy café in an industrial suburb. They were not permitted to have a bar, because the temptations of Demon Drink were still a spectre which haunted the mind of the college council; as a result, those who fell victim to it haunted the slightly squalid public houses in which the town abounded. The weaker members of the staff, on the other hand, who were hardly more favoured in the way of amenities, tended to drift into the bars of the town's more respectable hotels.

The wonder was that despite the visible and tangible neglect from which the students suffered, there was an almost total absence of what would today be called "student protest". They accepted almost without question the rule of primitive methodism imposed on them by the college administration. The reason was that the college, for all its inadequacies, did provide a genuine escape from the cramped material and intellectual conditions of the homes from which most of them came and the opportunity to enter a wider world than most of their fathers had known. What was sad was that their elders and teachers, instead of encouraging their appetite for freedom, did their best to confine them within the boundaries of the same narrow ethical and religious code which they had themselves inherited.

In this respect, Aberystwyth was unique even among the four colleges which together made up the University of Wales; certainly it would have been impossible to imagine a similar situation at any other British university at that time. But Aberystwyth, by reason of its geographical isolation from any large centre of population, had in many ways remained a backwater whose sluggish waters had not been stirred by the currents of the main stream of contemporary life; idols and shibboleths which had long been destroyed elsewhere here still preserved their original power. For the students, however, they were rapidly losing their virtue, and in this twilight of Methodist gods they tried to create a community of their own from which new life might spring. They accepted the prejudices of their elders with an easy and good-humoured indifference, almost, indeed, indulgence. They were far more innocent and unsophisticated than their counterparts at any English university, and they accepted almost without question the gerontocracy which ruled the college to an even greater extent than it rules most university institutions. But they were young, they were hopeful, and they were, I think, more intelligent than their English counterparts. To any kind of interest or encouragement they responded with an alacrity which was touching and affecting; and the very isolation in which they lived at Aberystwyth fostered among them a community of spirit, a reliance on their own efforts in creating their own forms of social intercourse, a sense that if they did not do these things for themselves nobody else would, which were admirable. They were the only truly living and vigorous element in the college and were as good material as any university institution could hope to find; and in the years which my wife and I spent at Aberystwyth they formed the only justification for the hopes which I had conceived when I first went there.

IV

This was over fifteen years ago and I have no doubt that in the interval things have changed very much for the better at Aberystwyth; it could hardly be possible that they should not. But when I arrived both the college and the town were in decay; they were like a house infected with dry rot which outwardly seems unchanged but is crumbling away within. So far as the college was concerned it was clear that many changes would have to be made, and some would have to be made quickly, which is never easy in any university; there had been an interregnum of a year since my predecessor had died, and many decisions had been postponed until a new principal had been appointed. There seemed to be skeletons in many cupboards, and they were only gradually revealed to me, sometimes with a certain *Schadenfreude* on the part of their curators at the thought that it was now my responsibility to dispose of them. At moments I had the impression that to dispose of skeletons was precisely what I had been called in for; only it was equally clear that there were many in the college, both on the staff and on the college council, to whom the skeletons were dear, like holy relics which should be treated with proper veneration. There were others who were equally determined that if any changes were to be made they should take a direction which conflicted sharply with all my ideas of what a university should be. Between them and myself the difference was in essence a very simple one, though in fact it showed itself in an extraordinarily wide variety of forms. I thought that a university could only have one single purpose, which is the pursuit of learning, either through teaching or research, and preferably through both; I equally thought an institution genuinely devoted to such a purpose could perform an invaluable service to Wales. But to others, who held their belief with a passionate intensity, learning was subsidiary, or should be, to the purpose of preserving Welsh culture and the Welsh language. At its simplest it was the difference between whether the college should be, or become, a university or a Welsh seminary.

I had been vaguely aware before arriving in Aberystwyth that there were some members of the college council who had strongly opposed my appointment, precisely on the ground that I did not have Welsh interests sufficiently at heart. Perhaps they were right, in the sense that I thought the interests of learning more important. I had not taken such opposition very seriously, though perhaps I should have when I was told by a friend at All Souls that he had been approached by a distinguished member of the council with an enquiry whether it was not true that I was a homosexual; the reason for the enquiry, it appeared, was my friendship with Guy, of which he had learned at the time of Guy's disappearance. Such a question seemed so absurd, to my friend as to myself, that I scarcely realized how deep a malice it concealed or to what lengths my opponents were willing to proceed.

I would have been wiser if I had understood that at Aberystwyth I was re-entering a society far more primitive than any which I had known for a very long time, in which nothing could be taken at its face value and everything had to be interpreted in terms of conflicts that were fought on some much lower level than the rational; it was something I had not encountered even in the lower depths of the army, though perhaps I should have reminded myself that in Germany I had seen how such forces can ruin and corrupt a great people. In the case of the college, I was exposed to the same atavistic instinct which wished to make of it an instrument shaped to achieve purely tribal ends and not an institution in which the light of reason might prevail. This instinct was all the stronger because the two forms in which Welsh tribal feeling had hitherto expressed itself most perfectly, language and religion, were in a process of rapid degeneration and decline. In my father's day a Methodist minister still commanded a greater prestige and respect than a professor; but now the minister preached to empty chapels while eager students clamoured for the privilege of listening to the professor; tribal feeling demanded that, religion failing, the professor should transmit the same ethical values as the minister had once preached. And my father had preached in Welsh, and now the Welsh language was also dying; tribal feeling demanded that in the university it should find a refuge in which it might arrest its decline and even recover a new strength. What was remarkable was that as Welsh culture lost its positive content, it expressed itself increasingly in an abstract nationalism in which fear and hatred played a larger part than love.

> *An intellectual hatred is the worst.*
> *Oh let her think opinions are accursed!*

says Yeats in his *A Prayer for my Daughter*. It was a prayer which I often felt like repeating at Aberystwyth.

Nationalism seemed to me necessarily hostile to the idea of a university, which unless wholly dedicated to the pursuit of knowledge, even when it threatens tribal idols, has lost its one single justification; without this, its functions are better performed by other institutions. Indeed, if the university were to be of any service to the Welsh people, and especially to the young students who had begun to win my affection, it could not do so by flattering their worst prejudices and their blindest instincts. I was prepared to say this publicly, and did so, and to apply it in the practical business of college administration; by doing so I earned the unremitting hostility of many of my Welsh colleagues, and it was all the fiercer because the support I found came in the main from English members of the staff, sad exiles in an alien land, for whom Welsh nationalism was an irritating irrelevance to the serious business of teaching and research.

It would perhaps be absurd to say that during the few years in which I remained at Aberystwyth the college became a battlefield between two diametrically opposed conceptions of what a university should be. To say so may seem to give too great an importance to what was happening in this obscure little corner of Cardiganshire. And yet the conflict made itself felt in almost every matter, important or trivial, which came up for discussion during my period as Principal. Inevitably, and primarily, of course, in the question of appointments; for which should come first in one's assessment of a candidate, his qualities as a scholar or as a Welshman? It made itself felt in the degree of liberty which should be permitted to students: for was the college really an institute of learning or a preceptor of Welsh morals? It affected the administration of the college's inadequate resources: should whatever there was to spare be devoted to departments which showed promise of making original contributions to learning, or to the provision of additional lecturers who would teach through the medium of Welsh? It even raised its head in the question of providing a community house for the academic staff; for if they had a house, would not its amenities include a bar, and would not a bar be in itself a betrayal of the Welsh Nonconformist ethic, and, even worse, would it not set a dangerous example to students? Most of all, the conflict entered into the question, none the less important because it could never be explicitly formulated, what kind of a person the Principal of the College should be? Should he be one who put the pursuit of knowledge above the preservation of the Welsh language, reason above Nonconformity, lowered his dignity by making friends with students and junior lecturers, was not greatly concerned with their morals as long as they did their work, and even helped to corrupt them by offering them a drink when he had invited them to his house?

In retrospect, I am sometimes amazed at, and ashamed of, the triviality of some of the issues which occupied so much of our time and thought at Aberystwyth, all given an unreal importance by the intrusion into the academic life of a principle of nationalism which was irrelevant to its proper purposes. It would be tedious, and certainly unedifying, to recount the number of occasions on which this permanent underlying issue made itself felt; but they gave to my few years as Principal of the college the character of a fierce and tenacious little war of attrition, enlivened by sudden sallies, patrol actions and commando raids, which both tried one's nerves and exhausted one's patience. It did not cause me the same kind of unhappiness which life at Aberystwyth caused my wife, because at least I had the satisfaction of thinking that I was trying to do something which was worth doing, while to her it seemed that both of us were wasting our lives; but certainly it made me wonder with increasing frequency whether this was the way in which I wished to live for ever.

My doubts were allayed because with time it began to seem that I and those who sympathized with my objects might even succeed in what we wished to do. Something of the gloom and stagnation which enveloped the college on my arrival began to lift. Something of the hierarchical stiffness which forbade professors to speak to senior lecturers, and senior lecturers to junior lecturers, and junior lecturers to students, and everyone to the Principal, was gradually relaxed. Skeletons became noticeably fewer in number. It sometimes became possible to discuss strictly academic subjects as if they were the real business of the college; it was even possible to relax or abolish some of the absurdly antiquated rules of discipline which were imposed on the students, and to persuade the college that young men and women of university age do not really benefit by being treated like school children. Sometimes I began to feel that we were really behaving as a university should; and sometimes we were even able to laugh at ourselves. I even began to hope that from this small college by the sea, in its magnificent natural setting, so thrown upon its own resources by its isolation from any large centres of population, something might emerge which would be an original and unique contribution to the university system, not only of Wales, but of the entire country.

Certainly there were good reasons for such a hope; I felt that given a good many more years of internecine warfare, of argument and persuasion, of innumerable committees in which, over and over again, nationalism and the Welsh language would continue to raise their King Charles's Heads, the college might become a place in which the genuine academic virtues would flourish. For really there was no reason why they should not. The students were only too willing and eager to learn from anyone who showed them sympathy and understanding, and if on occasions they voiced their dissatisfaction, they usually had good reason, and were entirely without that kind of destructive malice which has infected student protest today. Malice indeed was almost a monopoly of the senior staff, who manifested it impartially to each other, to myself, and to the students. Even this, however, was on the decline; many of the issues which most frequently and most bitterly provoked dissent were so obviously related to the past, so much a matter of tribal memory, that it was possible to hope that with time they would lose their emotive power.

Thus I was not without reason for confidence. There remained, however, a stubborn body of opinion in the college which, as the defender of what was called "the Welsh Way of Life", was unalterably hostile to the kind of policies I should have liked the college to adopt. Since I myself had described the Welsh way of life as that of a dying peasant culture which had its face resolutely turned to the past, I offered an obvious target for their hostility, and I suppose that, from their own point of view, they were right to see in me an enemy, though I found it difficult to believe that, most of all in a university, dis-agreements could be reduced to so personal a basis. It would have been difficult to define what they themselves meant by "the Welsh Way of Life" because so many different elements entered into it. For some, it was a matter entirely of the Welsh language, and for this they were willing to sacrifice any other interest. To some its essential quality was religious and ethical, and for them the college was, or should be, a kind of advanced version of a methodist Sunday school. To yet others, it was a question of nationalism and racialism, and for them the college was essentially an institution whose task was to train young men who would one day dedicate themselves to the cause of self-government for Wales. I found each of these aspects of the "Welsh Way of Life" equally antipathetic, and indeed even slightly absurd, and perhaps this was fortunate for my opponents, because their beliefs were in many respects incompatible with each other and they found it difficult to make common cause, as the Welsh so frequently do; in me, at least, they found someone to whom they were all equally opposed.

I do not know what would have happened if I had remained in Wales. I myself have the firm conviction that time was on my side, that my critics were all, in one respect or another, the defenders of lost causes, and that neither language, nor religion, nor nationalism would in the end prevail. But time precisely was what was not given me, and of this I cannot, and would not, wish to complain, because the occasion of my leaving Aberystwyth, for a second time, was entirely of my own making.

v

Once again, I find it difficult to analyse the obscure, complex motives which determined one's behaviour, and more especially when it is of a kind that changes one's whole life; and perhaps one ought to be all the more suspicious of them if, to oneself though not to others, they seem to be to one's credit.

The prospect of remaining for long at Aberystwyth, perhaps for the rest of my life, was not one which attracted me greatly. Indeed, I had not been there long before I began once again to feel stifled by that stale and claustrophobic air of Wales, in which ideas wither and die, and no issue is ever of any importance unless it has its roots deep in ancient memories; it was like the oppressive air of the little town huddled at the foot of the hills whose grey streets and mean conventicles seemed a fitting refuge for minds for which freedom was too dangerous an element into which to adventure. I told myself that I should not complain of this; after all I should have been forewarned and indeed had been repeatedly warned, by my brother, by my friends, that Wales was no place for me; if now I found my situation disagreeable I had only my own wilfulness to blame.

My dissatisfaction, however, was less important than my wife's unhappiness, which was intense. I was acutely aware that it was entirely due to me that she found herself an exile on this Celtic fringe of Britain, whose manners and customs were entirely foreign to her, its language unintelligible and its inhabitants hostile. Even the roses that bloomed at Christmas, the garden she had made for herself where everything grew in a wild profusion that was only accentuated by the grim austerity of the botanical beds, the little owl that perched at night on the edge of the path through the woods, did not comfort her; much as she loved her plants and her flowers, they could not make up for the absence of recognizable human beings, which to her the Welsh were not.

Her unhappiness made for mine, though I am ashamed to say that my own behaviour at that particular time only increased her misery and loneliness. Perhaps, in the depths of my mind, or whatever it is that really determines one's actions, there was a sense that only some particularly flagrant act of folly could bring to an end a situation which was rapidly becoming intolerable; perhaps I was only obeying an instinct for self-destruction which my wife herself regarded as particularly Welsh. But if such motives entered into my behaviour I was unaware of them; strangely enough, I thought I was behaving rationally. However that may be, there was perhaps a kind of rough justice in the fact that the provocation to action originated, certainly without any intention on his part, with Guy.

Since returning to Aberystwyth, I had not thought a great deal about him. My life in Wales, from which either London or Oxford or Cambridge seemed at times infinitely remote, was so completely detached from everything, either serious or trivial, which had ever joined us together that at times I found it almost difficult to believe that he had ever existed. It was rather as if, living at the North Pole, one had tried to remember that once one had lived on the Equator. And if he had ever existed, it was by now at least doubtful whether he still did. In its White Paper the government had said as little as it could about the mystery of his and Maclean's disappearance, in the hope, perhaps, that public interest in the case would die from lack of information; it had caused serious damage to Anglo-American relations and in the government's view the sooner it was forgotten the better. None of the enquiries indefatigably pursued by the Press had given the slightest clue to Guy's whereabouts, or indeed to whether he was still alive, though by then the most reasonable assumption was that both he and Maclean were in the Soviet Union.

If that were indeed the case, I myself felt that it were better if he were dead. For him, of all people, deprived of everything which he liked most, I could foresee nothing but a long-drawn-out disintegration in the Socialist Fatherland; the kind of adaptation required for an exile to make himself at home in a foreign country was beyond his powers. Yet somehow I knew perfectly well that he was alive; it was impossible that his grotesquely vivid nature should so abruptly have ceased to exist, even in the world of melodrama which he had chosen to enter. And equally I was convinced that if he were still alive, we had not heard the last of him, and that his disappearance would have further consequences.

For me, amid all my other preoccupations at Aberystwyth, he existed in a kind of limbo of the memory, a ghost on whom it was still possible to suspend judgement until one knew exactly how and why he had been removed from the land of the living. Despite all the trouble and distress he had caused to so many who had been his friends, I still retained my affection for him and continued to remember him as part of the world of my youth in which, strangely enough, I had been, despite all the terrible events which had led it to disaster, intensely happy. It seemed the best way to remember him; I had the feeling that if he were to reappear, the results might be exceedingly unpleasant. And so they were, and particularly for myself, though this was entirely my own fault.

On Saturday, February 11th, 1956, in the National Hotel in Moscow, Guy Burgess and Donald Maclean appeared before a hastily summoned Press conference, apparently in good health and spirits, handed out prepared statements and left. The statements left no doubt that they were indeed, and had been, communists and communist agents and that they had chosen to live in the Socialist Fatherland to which all their adult lives had been dedicated.

I find it difficult to account for the effect which their reappearance, and the public statements which accompanied it, made upon me. They were like some chilly official announcement that every suspicion I had ever had of Guy had been correct and that all the theories, excuses, explanations, which I had found or invented in order to exorcise them, had been merely self-deceptions practised in order to conceal the truth from myself. It seemed extraordinary to realize at last that Guy had in fact told me the truth, and that for nearly twenty years I had *known* that Guy was a Soviet agent but had been unable to acknowledge the fact; or had I, and merely evaded the issue?

The truth, at last, plain and unvarnished, was difficult to accept. Especially because, as a result, many people had suffered, some perhaps in ways I did not like to think of. It was equally difficult to accept that for all those years Guy, apart from his one single moment of self-revelation, had consciously and consistently betrayed all the affection which his friends had had for him, in spite of all the strains to which he had so often exposed it. I seemed to see Guy in a new light, as if someone in whom, for all his faults, one had recognized a kind of virtue, had been suddenly revealed in a character which belonged to a different mental and emotional world from oneself.

I do not know whether such feelings were justified. I suppose that it was still possible to make out a case for admiring Guy and what he had done; that is to say, as one who had committed himself so completely to a cause that he had not hesitated to sacrifice to it both himself and his friends. And indeed, in Guy's case, the extent of the sacrifice was so great that it might well inspire admiration. Unfortunately, in the years since the great Soviet state trials and the conclusion of the German-Soviet pact, I had come to look upon the cause for which the sacrifice had been made as no less ignoble than the methods which it used to promote its own ends; among which, by now, it was clear that one should include Guy's own activities.

It is perhaps not necessary to explain here the process of disillusion by which one comes to see a cause in which one has placed one's highest hopes as an embodiment of evil. Others have done it better than I can; the story of *The God That Failed* is one of the fundamental stories of my generation and it has been told in so many different versions during the last thirty years that my own version of it would add nothing to the others. It is perhaps enough to say that, far from seeing Guy as one who had sacrificed himself for higher ends, I saw him as one who had advanced an unworthy cause by equally unworthy means. Even more, he had become in my eyes one who had voluntarily engaged in the cruel and murderous operations of an organization which was directly responsible for the destruction of millions of people by death, torture, starvation and any other means which its ingenuity could devise to achieve that purpose. He was, no doubt, my friend; he was also a man with blood on his hands.

It might be said that I should have realized this before. The point was that I had not known it with certainty and that, in such a case, only certainty could justify one in passing judgement. On grounds of friendship I had for as long as possible made every reservation I could which would offer any explanation for Guy's conduct except the true one. In doing so, it seemed to me, I had to some extent made myself his accomplice; some of the blood had rubbed off on me.

Perhaps I was over-sensitive to feel in this way; but the guilt I felt in regard to Guy and my dealings with him was exacerbated by a more general sense of guilt which was inspired by the support and approval which, in the 30s and even later, I had given to the Communist party of the Soviet Union. Indeed, in my attitude to the Soviet Union I had behaved in much the same way as I had to Guy; that is to say that, even after I had sufficient evidence to recognize it for what it was, I had continued to make

every kind of reservation and excuse for its conduct,
however evil its consequences might be.

It would perhaps have been easy to forgive oneself on
the grounds that one had been under the spell of an
illusion to which thousands of others had also fallen a
victim; one always finds it easy to forgive oneself. But in
this case it was not merely a matter of forgiveness. It was
also a matter, as it seemed to me, of trying to limit the
amount of harm one had done, even if, in relation to the
monstrous evils for which the Communist party had been
responsible, one's own contribution to them had been so
minute as to mean nothing, except perhaps to oneself.
There are situations to which a moral calculus of this
kind hardly seems relevant. I felt something of that wholly
irrational sense which involuntarily recurred to Rubashov
in Arthur Koestler's *Darkness at Noon* and which he
expressed in the almost meaningless words: *I must pay.*

There is something absurd about such a comparison;
and indeed I was sharply aware that my own feelings were
absurd. Yet it seemed to me that there was something
very simple I could do which might give some rational
meaning to them; this was to tell the truth about my
relations with Guy, and what one had learned as a result,
as simply and truthfully as possible. At the time of his
disappearance I felt that I had already discharged this
responsibility by making my statement to MI5. Yet I was
haunted by the suspicion that, for a variety of reasons,
MI5 was inhibited from making any effective use of any
information which I gave them; as later events showed,
the suspicion was not unjustified. I remained convinced
that Guy and Maclean had not operated alone, that others
remained to continue their work, and that the likeliest
place to look for them was in the security services themselves. In telling MI5 my story, was I not simply ensuring

that it would fall into hands which had every interest in suppressing it?

Quis enim custodet custodes? If the security services themselves were not to be trusted, in whom could one securely place one's trust? I felt that I had become involved in a world of subterfuges and deceptions in which nothing was what it seemed; it was like one of those nightmares in which faces, masks, grinning images continually shift and dissolve to reveal yet other shapes behind them and there was also the sense that at the end of the nightmare's long corridors there lay the very real flesh and blood horrors for which Guy's masters were responsible, and through them reverberated the shrieks in the night of their victims.

These may seem strange thoughts to obsess the mind of the Principal of a small Welsh university college, safely removed from such horrors in the pastoral landscape of Cardiganshire. And no doubt, for a variety of reasons a certain element of the higher lunacy entered into them; this particular nightmare had, in a variety of forms, pursued me for so long, and with increasing intensity, that its subjective and objective aspects had become inextricably confused and I felt that only by some violent effort could I be rid of it.

There was, I thought, only one thing I could do, and that was to write down what I knew as accurately as I could, while taking into account all the doubts, hesitations, suspicions that had led me to behave as I had. I did not know that it would serve any very useful purpose, but at least it might help to put my own mind at rest. Yet there remained the conviction that the story of Guy and Maclean had not yet come to an end and that there were still developments to come which for some people might prove serious. If that were so, it seemed best that, so far as it was in my power, everyone concerned should be forewarned.

I did not think that my own account would do me very much credit. At best I would look foolish, perhaps absurd, and at worst tainted by my association with Guy. And to some, I knew, the mere act of committing to paper what I knew about him would be regarded as treacherous and dishonourable. I did not much look forward to such consequences but in the end, I thought, to tell the truth was the only alternative left to me. *Magna est veritas et praevalebit;* it was with some such naive slogan in my mind that I sat down and rapidly wrote the account of my relations with Guy which, with only minor changes, forms the substance of the third and fourth sections of this book.

There remained the question of what was to be done with the manuscript. I had not written it merely for the record; I wished it to be published, both as an account of the circumstances, so far as I knew them, which had led up to Guy's disappearance and as a kind of warning that his activities as a Soviet agent might be expected to have further consequences. I accordingly dispatched the manuscript to my literary agents, who were wise enough to warn me that publication might give rise to some scandal; when I replied that I was aware of this, but nevertheless wished to proceed, they arranged for publication, in six consecutive articles, in the *People*, a Sunday newspaper which felt that their material was sensational enough to appeal to its mass audience. The articles were to be based on the material contained in my manuscript but were to be written by a member of the *People's* staff, in a style which they felt would be more acceptable to their readers than my own, and would therefore appear anonymously. I had some doubts about the wisdom of this arrangement, but I felt that I was now committed to pursue the matter to the end whatever the consequences, and therefore gave my agreement.

VI

My literary agent had certainly not exaggerated in saying that the appearance of the articles might have unfortunate consequences; they were indeed far worse than anything I had foreseen. In one respect, however, they achieved, in part at least, the object which I had intended; for among their earliest readers were MI5, who immediately dispatched two officers to Aberystwyth, with a request for a copy of my original manuscript; they read it with almost microscopic attention and interrogated me closely about every detail of its contents. Somehow they gave me the impression that, in the interval since Guy's and Maclean's disappearance, and perhaps as a result of it, there had been considerable changes in their organization and that, though my manuscript did not materially differ from my original statement to them, they were now prepared to pay rather more serious attention to what I had to say.

But it was not only MI5 who were interested in the articles, especially because their anonymity was not preserved for long, and a gossip columnist in the *Daily Telegraph* revealed that their author was the Principal of the University College of Wales. Even in the wider world the announcement created considerable interest; in Aberystwyth, and in the college, it had something of the effect of the bombardment of Fort Sumter in provoking the American Civil War. Nor perhaps was this surprising for the *People* had rewritten and edited my manuscript so as the achieve the most sensational possible effect. The result was such as to give my critics, both within and without the college, a scarcely hoped for opportunity to rid themselves of one whom they regarded as a renegade Welshman intent on destroying everything which they held most dear. It is almost impossible to dismiss the Principal of a college, once he has been duly appointed, except on grounds of flagrant immorality or neglect of duty, and even publishing articles in the sensational Sunday press could hardly be held to fall into either of these two categories. But it is possible, given sufficient determination and malice, to make life so unpleasant for him as to make his position untenable, and even, by innuendo and insinuation, to hint that his past has been stained by unnameable vices.

To this task my critics applied themselves with a vigour and virtuosity which were worthy of a better cause, and with such success that in Wales the affair of the articles quickly assumed the proportions of a national scandal, so grave indeed that I was politely informed by the President of the college, a distinguished lawyer of impeccable virtue, a dull mind, and ardent Welsh patriotism, that he had no alternative but to ask for my resignation. He was, however, prepared to do a deal; that is to say, if I were to go quickly, quietly and without resistance, he was prepared to make my departure as easy for me as possible.

I was not, however, prepared to resign; it seemed to me that it would not be for the good of myself nor, in the long run, of the college, and I was reluctant to abandon my friends on the staff and on the council who were in sympathy with my ideas for reforming it. Nor indeed did I believe that my position as its Principal in any way precluded me from writing and publishing whatever I liked and in whatever manner I pleased. My refusal to resign required that less diplomatic means of attack should be adopted; at the next meeting of the college council, a resolution was proposed that a committee should be set up to enquire into my conduct in writing and publishing the articles. I opposed the resolution and it was defeated, and with a sense that a storm had subsided in a tea-cup, I left Aberystwyth with my wife and family to spend a holiday on the marvellous estuary of the Mawddach in North Wales.

I should not have been deceived by so easy a victory, and within a few days I was summoned back to Aberystwyth, to attend an emergency meeting of the council, summoned by the President in response to a demand by twelve professors that a committee of enquiry be appointed. When I returned the atmosphere of the little town was something between that of a fairground and a public execution; the streets were crowded with farmers in for market, newspaper placards announced the summoning of the council, and members of the Press and eager sightseers crowded the precincts of the college and the bars of its hotels and public houses.

On this occasion I did not feel I could resist the demand for an enquiry, but I repeated my belief that it could serve no purpose, as there could be no possible subject of investigation except the articles themselves, and as these had already been studied with microscopic attention by the entire population of Wales, I did not feel that the committee could add anything further to them. I was of course mistaken, as indeed I was at every stage of this strange little drama; in the course of it I came to realize, as I should have realized before, that common sense and practical judgement are qualities with which perhaps I am not conspicuously endowed.

The committee, when it was at length constituted, consisted of three gentlemen of impeccable social, professional and academic credentials; they were all English, because it was felt that the passions of Welshmen were so deeply engaged that an impartial judgement could not be expected of them. It had not been easy to constitute the committee; a long list of eminent persons had to be approached before three could be found who were willing to undertake the disagreeable commission with which they were entrusted. Once appointed, however, the committee set about its task with a thoroughness and a zest which protracted their proceedings over a period of some eight months. I and other members of the college staff were summoned to appear before them in London; my own interview consisted of a lengthy and unmistakeably hostile cross-examination by the chairman, who appeared to consider that his terms of reference included any possible aspect of my public or private life which might be open to criticism. A devout Anglican, he could not conceal his horror that Guy should have been a godfather to one of my two sons; in fact, Guy could not have been a kinder or more affectionate one. The Vice-Principal of the college, a distinguished physicist who throughout my troubles behaved to me both as a friend and as the most loyal of colleagues, was handled with almost equal severity and subjected to an inquisition to show that, with my connivance, he had failed to maintain proper discipline among the students; for such a suggestion there was not the slightest evidence, except the exemplary tolerance and understanding with which he had administered the almost medieval rules of discipline which obtained in the college.

Having completed its enquiries in London, the committee proceeded to visit Aberystwyth, where it sat for three days taking evidence from anyone who wished to offer himself, or herself, as a witness. They were many,

because the committee's procedure permitted every kind
of allegation, however false or irrelevant, to be made
about me; many strange bees escaped from many Welsh
bonnets. A sympathetic member of the college council
found it necessary to warn me that I was charged, among
other things, with homosexuality, with hostility to Welsh
nationalist aspirations, and with corrupting students by
offering them a glass of sherry when they visited us;
it was not clear which was the most serious of these
charges.

It had by now become clear to me that the committee
was conducting, not an enquiry, but a prosecution. This
became even clearer when, in reply to my request that I
should be told what offences I was charged with, and
shown the evidence on which they were based, the committee refused on the grounds that this was not customary
in an enquiry of a disciplinary nature. But the committee's
attitude also revealed to me something which I had not
hitherto understood, which was that by publishing the
articles in the *People*, I had, at one stroke, simultaneously
succeeded in giving offence not only to the Welsh, but
also to the English Establishment. That the Welsh
should be offended was perhaps not surprising; the
articles had simply confirmed their feeling that I was not
the man required to fill the honoured position of Principal
of the University College of Wales, a national institution
of which Wales was proud. To the English Establishment, however, the articles were a breach of that complicated moral code by which it is held together, and most
of all of those personal loyalties to which it gives an almost
religious value. They were worse than a moral trans-
gression; they were an act of bad taste, which tended to
throw an unpleasant light on the *sacra arcana* of the
English Establishment.

My sense that I had committed a double offence, against good taste and decent feeling, was confirmed by letters and protests which I began to receive soon after the first of the articles was published. The warden of an Oxford college, for whom I felt an affection which dated from my undergraduate days, wrote to suggest that I should plant a screen of Judas trees around the college athletic fields. A distinguished moral philosopher, also an old friend, was shocked, not by the content of the articles, but by the fact that they had appeared in so vulgar and sensational a paper as the *People*; in some more reputable journal, they might even have had some literary value. In the *People* they were unforgivable. Such a letter seemed to me to reveal an almost classical confusion of moral and aesthetic values, reducing both to triviality; moral indignation of such a kind seemed to spring from singularly impure sources. It was perhaps hardly worth more than the reaction of a literary lady with whom I was to dine in London who hurriedly cancelled the invitation on the ground that my presence would give offence to her other guests; I was no longer, as the Germans would say, *salonfähig*.

I was, it seemed, in disgrace not only with my Welsh critics but with my English friends, except however for some few, like Louis McNeice, John Sparrow, R. C. Zaehner, A. J. Ayer, F. W. Deakin, Douglas Young and David Footman, who continued to show me the same affection as before; I record their names out of gratitude for the sympathy and understanding which they showed during the worst of my troubles. I even discovered new friends, both in England and in Wales, who encouraged me to believe that the disapproval provoked by the articles was purely ephemeral and that with time it would disappear and my tribulations would be over.

I found it difficult to believe that they were right. The articles had provoked such violent feelings that I felt they had destroyed any further usefulness I might have at Aberystwyth; Welshmen have the most tenacious of memories, especially for scandal, and I knew that for many years to come the articles would remain a cause of controversy both within the college and outside it. In any case, they had already provoked so many manifestations of malice and hostility, so many shabby manœuvres, so much rancour and gossip, that I knew I could never again make my home in Aberystwyth; my feeling was all the stronger because gossip spared my wife and children no more than myself. To my wife this was only another addition to the unhappiness she had felt almost as soon as she had taken up residence in Aberystwyth; to my children, however, it was something entirely new to find themselves, in the local schools which they then attended, the victims of the malice which their school-fellows had learned from their parents.

As the months went by, and the committee continued its apparently interminable researches, I decided both that it was impossible, and that I did not wish, to continue as Principal of the college. It seemed to me clear, from the wholly partisan spirit in which the committee had pursued its enquiries, that I could expect nothing from its report which would be likely to make me change my mind, for it was indefatigable in investigating the slightest innuendo or insinuation that had been made against me. Whether it believed them or not, its procedure tended to give them an importance which they would otherwise have wholly lacked. The mere fact that presumably serious and intelligent men should think them worth listening to seemed to endow them with significance. That they should travel to Aberystwyth to ensure that not even the most trivial item of gossip should go unheard seemed in itself evidence of the importance they attached to it.

After these mountainous labours, their report emerged as a vicious little mouse. They reviewed, without indicating their sources, the evidence that had been laid before them, and concluded that they could find no ground for criticism in it either of myself personally or of my conduct of the college's affairs; indeed, in this latter respect, they conceded somewhat reluctantly, that they had been conducted very well and to the benefit of the college. The articles, however, they condemned as a "lewd document", a phrase so heavy with moral and legal implications that it was in itself sufficient to indicate their belief that I was not a proper person to be Principal of the college. They took an even worse view, however, of my own manuscript, on which the articles had originally been based. Their moral susceptibilities were offended both by the fact that I had written it and, almost worse, that my wife had typed it for me. The report implied that my wife had connived at some particularly distasteful form of literary obscenity.

The report was certainly not calculated to alter my decision to resign my appointment and immediately I received it I informed the college of my intention. My friends in the college pressed me to stay; the students, in particular, demonstrated in every way open to them their wish that I should remain. But a college, or a university, is essentially a community which depends on the mutual trust and confidence that exists between all its members and I was well aware that, by my own action, I had provoked far too much criticism and antagonism for good relations within the college to be easily restored. If I remained, it was inevitable that the college would divide into two bitterly hostile factions, and I was sure that such a situation was one in which neither the college nor I would prosper. The atmosphere of the college meeting at which I insisted that my resignation be received was in itself sufficient evidence of this; it was bitter and acrimonious and revived once again all the old animosities which had plagued the college since my arrival. It was perhaps some small satisfaction that the college refused to approve the committee's report but merely recorded its reception.

On the morning after the college meeting I left Aberystwyth, leaving my family behind. The future seemed bleak in the extreme. At the age of forty-five, with a wife and five young children to support, I found myself homeless, without visible means of subsistence, unemployed and, in any academic capacity, henceforth virtually unemployable. Even so, as I stood on the platform at Aberystwyth's grim little railway station, waiting for the train to carry me on the nine-hour journey to London, I could not repress a sense of happiness and liberation at this second escape from my birthplace.

A month later I was run over by a Volkswagen mini-bus at Littlewick Green, on the road between Reading and Maidenhead, and, I suppose, came as near to death as it is possible without actually dying. I suffered multiple injuries and severe concussion, and for some time it was thought unlikely that I would recover. When, after several weeks, I regained consciousness it was like being born again, but into a world which was very different from anything I had ever known before.

ABOUT THE AUTHOR

GORONWY REES, who has been a novelist, soldier, educator, and journalist, is one of the leading intellectual personalities in England today. He was born in Wales in 1909, and was educated in Cardiff and at New College, Oxford. Before the outbreak of World War II, he was a leader writer on the *Manchester Guardian* and an assistant editor of *The Spectator*. During the War he was commissioned an officer in the Royal Welch Fusiliers. As a Fellow of All Souls he returned to Oxford as the Estates Bursar, and after that took up an appointment as the Principal of University College of Wales in Aberystwyth (1953-1957). Among his books are a study of *The Multi-Millionaires,* a history of *The Rhine* and a collection of essays entitled *A Bundle of Sensations.* His three novels are: *A Summer Flood, A Bridge to Divide Them,* and *Where No Wounds Were.* He is also well-known as a translator: Büchner's *Danton's Death* (with Stephen Spender), and the forthcoming new edition of Janouch's *Conversations with Kafka.* In recent years he has been writing a regular column for *Encounter,* the London literary monthly, under "R." He lives in London, is married, and is the father of three sons and two daughters.